# EASY FITNESS FOR OVER FORTIES

*Your Fitness Plan For Life*

Chris Morris

YOU'VE GOT TO EXERCISE. YOUR HEALTH ACCOUNT, YOUR
BANK ACCOUNT, THEY'RE THE SAME THING. THE MORE
YOU PUT IN, THE MORE YOU CAN TAKE OUT.
—JACK LALANNE

# CONTENTS

# PREFACE

Several years ago I realized that I was in serious danger of becoming much older than my years. It was a time when I seemed inexorably to be putting on the pounds, leading a largely sedentary lifestyle in front of a computer while eating and drinking far too much.

It was driven home to me during a family holiday which seemed mostly to involve climbing hills to and from a hotel which, due to bad planning on my part, was positioned on top of a hill overlooking the town. Watching my family disappear upwards as I made slow progress back to the hotel really opened my eyes to how unfit I had become. They did stop and wait for the oldie from time to time, of course! In my fast-encroaching middle age, fitness seemed a thing of the past, something which I could no longer hope to attain.

**But What To Do About It?**

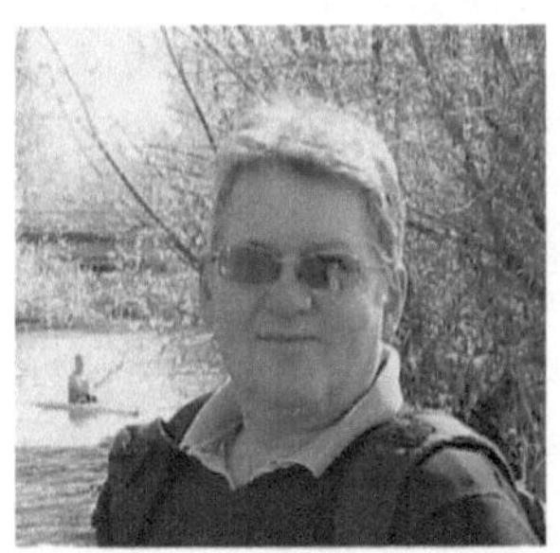

However, I am quite stubborn at times, and this was one of them. So on my return home, I approached the scales with trepidation. Knowing that I was overweight, but still expecting to be weighing in at around 170 pounds - or maybe just a little bit more - I was horrified to find that I was even heavier than my worst imaginings. Around 30 pounds heavier than my younger weight, and far, far too much for my height. No wonder I was finding hills difficult, carrying all those extra pounds!

It's not all about weight, of course. I realized that regular exercise was something I was lacking, and would be the key to being as fit as I aspired to be. Losing weight would just be a by-product of being fit.

And so it proved.

**The Secret**

There is no single secret. I tried different combinations of exercises and a more careful diet, writing down everything I was eating and drinking and what exercise I was doing. Less than three months later, after hitting on just the right balance of exercise that wouldn't disrupt my busy life, I was feeling as fit as I had done for many years. On vacation, with over 20 pounds shed, it was a pleasure not to be walking around at the poolside vainly trying to hold in a flabby belly.

But losing that (relatively small) amount of weight doesn't reveal the true story. Because weight - in itself - is irrelevant. It is how you carry yourself, your muscle tone, confidence in yourself along with a certain 'bouncy fitness', all these things and more, which are the true, long-lasting benefits of the program I now follow. Watching the scales is a distraction, because you know, in yourself, how fit you feel. I feel – and look -much fitter than before (compare the two pictures), and I am no longer simply 'over 40', but 'over 60' too.

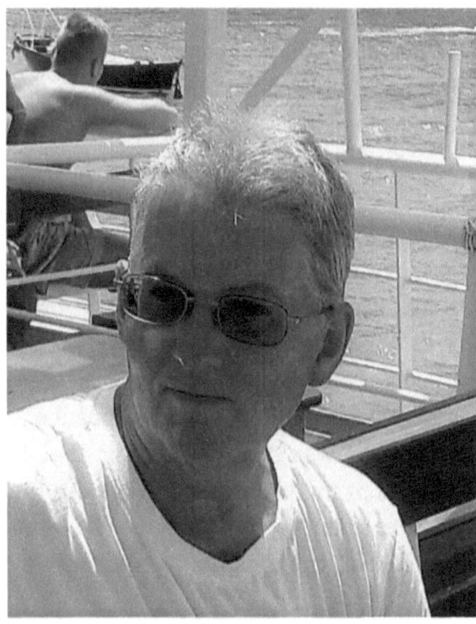

**Fitness on demand**

I have refined and fine-tuned my program over the last few years, to the point where I now have fitness at my command. Put on a pound or three after a period of over-indulgence and little activity, and I feel lethargic. All I need to do is to step up the easy fitness program for two or three days and the fitness level is back.

Not super-fit, and definitely no obsessive body-building or hyper-activity. Just a steady, constant fitness without having to change my whole lifestyle. I still enjoy beer, wine, burgers, whatever may be considered to be 'bad for you'. The key is to enjoy everything in moderation. No need to give up the things you enjoy. Maintaining fitness while leading an enjoyable lifestyle as I head into older age is the aim – and the achievement.

## Now, what about you?

# INTRODUCTION

Welcome to your first day of *Easy Fitness for Over 40s*. I named the program 'Easy' because I originally designed it for myself and I like things easy. And there's no other word for it, because that's exactly what it is.

The entire 'Easy' program is built around a sequence of easy daily exercise routines, combined with regular secondary exercise. Sitting around for hours a day is often inevitable - at your workplace, travelling, even surfing the net - but actively planning to be active when you can will make all the difference. In our grandparents' day being active for much of the day was often a necessity. In modern times we have the luxury of being able to make a choice.

There is also a third element to this program, which is a subtle shift towards a healthier lifestyle. This includes diet (but not diet*ing*) as well as physical and mental wellbeing.

Through the course of this book you will develop in just 12 weeks into a vastly improved version of your current self. Someone who will draw complimentary remarks from your friends. Stick with it, and it will happen.

Underlying the whole series of *Easy Fitness* programs is a philosophy of recognizing that heading into middle age and older age is inevitably drawing closer, so you may as well prepare properly for when you arrive there. Nobody wants to be unhealthy and housebound as we grow older, and a change of lifestyle **now** is as good a time as any to safeguard your future.

An important strand of the *Easy Fitness* philosophy is to be able to enjoy life - and good health - on your own terms, without having to give up many of the things which you may find enjoyable. A good diet is a good thing, but not to the exclusion of a few regular treats along the way. Moderation over self-denial.

Obviously I can make no promise about your future health, because I don't know you, nor do I know your current level of fitness or medical needs. What I do know, however, is that becoming fit and staying fit is a fundamental aspect of living a longer and healthier life.

The exercise routines will take 15-20 minutes to complete, depending on what fitness level you are at right now and how quickly you develop as you progress through the program. At every stage you reach you will definitely be aware that you have put in some effort, because every worthwhile exercise needs to be challenging to some extent, but you should never find yourself having to push through any 'pain barrier'.

The biggest challenge of all is to start. That takes a degree of motivation to overcome an ongoing reluctance to take action, but you have already shown some motivation in getting this far, on the cusp of a new, fitter you. I will show you how to gain all the motivation you need to finish this program later on.

When you arrive at an optimized fitness level then you will be able to take all the exercises in your stride and need far less motivation to keep up the momentum. After you have seen the results, why would you not want to spend 15 or 20 minutes of your day to maintain that newly enhanced body?

I myself can do all the exercises to the maximum recommended level without any significant effort at all, and you are probably a relative spring chicken compared to a grizzly old bird like me. In fact I often complete a few more routines just because I feel like it and really enjoy it when I'm in the mood. Sometimes it's almost as easy to keep going as to stop!

The most important message I want to pass on to you at this introductory phase is that you must complete every one of the exercise routines set out below, on a regular basis and to the best of your capability. If you make excuses then none of this will be truly worth doing, and you will probably never get to experience the best aspect of all - achieving a transcendent level where exercise becomes so *easy* that it is second nature. A new habit.

In fact exercise can become such a habit that whenever you may need to go into hyper-drive every now and then - which I find that life's demands occasionally call for - by stepping up to my Easy Extreme program it is possible to add muscle tone and lose weight very quickly. Going on vacation for example, who doesn't want to arrive with a healthy posture, fluid movement and a positive vitality that will shine through everything you do? Once you have mastered this program, it becomes easy to do exactly that on demand, whether you want to look good for a brand-new job, or simply to rejuvenate yourself after a celebratory blow-out. No need to feel jaded as long as you have the necessary foundation of fitness that I will be showing you over the following pages.

# THE FIRST STEP: COMMITTING TO YOUR FUTURE

Let's start with one of the most important keys to your success in becoming fitter in your forties. This is the foundation which will keep you motivated to continue whenever you feel that doing nothing is the easier option. It shouldn't happen too often, because as I always stress, these exercises really are easy.

Nevertheless, there will be times when you may feel that you just can't be bothered to make the effort. Mainly at the beginning, because the exercises may be unfamiliar, and seem more difficult than they really are. Then a little later, after one or two weeks, you may look at yourself and think - "I haven't lost much weight yet, I look just the same, it's not worthwhile, may as well give up." Please, please don't fall into that trap, because you will be missing out on the great benefits which are just about to happen, probably within the following few days.

Here is what you should do to guard against that inner voice. You need to do this before you do anything else. I know you want to be fitter, and all the things which come with that.

But the real question is what, exactly, will being fitter mean to you? Is it mainly because you still want to look good in the clothes which may not fit you quite as well as they did when you bought them? Is it because you feel that your age is catching up with you, and the activities which seemed so much easier just a few years ago are now becoming a great effort? Is it because you want to carry on being strong, healthy and still cut a good figure as you mature? Possibly all of them, or something different entirely.

Your motivation for wanting to become fit is individual to you, and that means you should define in your own mind what you really want to be able to gain through greater fitness. This is your personal 'grand vision'.

Try to see in your mind's eye the body image you aspire to. It may help if you imagine the style of clothes that you feel you can't wear right now, but would dearly love to. A drop in size may help, a return to your more youthful body shape. You may feel that a drop in weight is a good target to aim for, but try to visualize it, rather than seeing it as just a number. Weight doesn't necessarily 'fall off' simply through exercising, but fat certainly can. You will know when you feel and look good, even if the scales don't necessarily reflect that. You may also have some more physical ambition, such as being able to walk up some steep hills in your local area without struggling for breath, or something more challenging like being able to run a half-marathon.

Be as specific as possible, write it down and refer to it daily. You could fill in the space below if you have a printed copy of this book, because you will be coming back here quite a lot over the next few weeks.

*(Complete your **grand vision** with as much detail as you can, and replace the suggestions with your own goals if you prefer.)*

*I want to be*................................................................................................................

................................................................................................................

................................................................................................................

................................................................................................................

................................................................................................................

*I want to look like*................................................................................................

................................................................................................................

................................................................................................................

................................................................................................................

*I want to weigh*................................................................................................

*I am going to*........................................................................................................................

........................................................................................................................................

........................................................................................................................................

........................................................................................................................................

........................................................................................................................................

Challenge yourself, be aspirational, but also be realistic. It's a worthwhile ambition to improve your physique and elements of your body shape, but in truth you won't be able to fundamentally alter the body you were born with. Your genes may be fixed, but whether you can fit *into* your jeans is not. That *is* under your control, as you will be learning more about later on.

The next step is vital. You should nominate a fixed date to focus on for achieving your grand vision. It doesn't matter if it is six months from now, two years from now, or even longer. Just write it down and we will work towards that target together.

You may now be thinking that all this is just fantasy, that it isn't going to happen just by writing things down. The truth is, if you hold on to those thoughts then they won't.

On the other hand, if you have an end goal in sight all the time then you can measure your progress as you begin to get there in incremental stages, however small. The snowball effect will kick in as you gain momentum, and what once seemed a far off prospect will become within reach at an increasing pace.

At this stage you really need a fixed idea, a fixed date and a sense of determination to make something happen. It is important to grasp that although the exercises you will be doing are 'easy', there will be times when you need to push yourself to do them. The motivation to persevere when you would really prefer to give them a miss, 'just for today', comes from keeping your end goal in sight at all times.

At first you may feel inclined not to bother because you are not seeing instant results. This is very common. Your end goal, the grand vision, must be powerful enough to drive you on, to prevent you from taking the easy way out.

Have faith that you really will accomplish what you first set out to do. It really will happen, but you know the phrase about leading a horse to water. I can take you there over the rest of this book and accompany you on your journey. I can show you how to make progress in your journey, but you must have confidence that your journey's end will bring the results that you desire.

The best part is that you will find 'easy fitness' becoming easier and easier very quickly. After just 20 - 30 days you will find that the exercises have become a habit, that the routines become routine, slotting naturally into your day.

From then on, your journey towards your end goal will become easier, and your improvement will be noticeable for anyone to see, a source of pride.

## *Tell Someone*

Tell a member of your close circle what you are planning to do. You don't have to tell them all the intimate details of your long-term vision, but if you tell someone about your ambition for improved fitness you can count on their support and encouragement at times when your resolve is weakening.

This makes for an extra boost in your resolve, a drive to demonstrate to that person that you really can do it.

That is the First Step completed. In the next phase we will get down to the nitty gritty.

# THE SECOND STEP: MAKING IT ALL HAPPEN

There is an elephant in the room, and its name is procrastination. Right now, your personal end goal probably seems a distant dream.

Just like New Year resolutions, we usually launch into them with really good intentions, and then life inevitably gets in the way. One day slips by, then another a few days later, and before we know it our best laid plans have fallen by the wayside.

This is true of most long-term plans. It is all too easy to delay starting, or skip a day before getting any momentum going, because the end goal is so far on the horizon that it's almost out of sight.

December seems a long way off in January, and the inclination can all too easily be to put things off for a while. Suddenly it's September and the once-distant deadline now seems alarmingly close. With that alarm comes a sense of overwhelm. Then there's a rush to the 'finishing line' in a panic to achieve as much as possible before it's too late. Will that result in as great an achievement as that gained by a better structured approach? I don't think so.

To avoid such a haphazard scenario my advice is to deconstruct a goal into its primary elements and then to rebuild them into a series of targets lasting just 12 weeks. Each 12-week target leads progressively towards the end goal, which may be 6 months, 12 months or even further away.

During each individual phase you can reinforce to yourself the mantra that "in just 12 weeks from now I will have achieved something really special." A measurable improvement that represents an important milestone on the road to your end goal, your grand vision.

A 12-week period concentrates your efforts incredibly effectively. It is just long enough to accomplish some feat that is really significant. Yet at the same time, its duration is short enough to make its end point reassuringly close.

Your exercise plan takes full advantage of this mind-focusing yardstick which is founded on some of the life-changing concepts developed in the stimulating book *The Twelve Week Year* by Brian P. Moran and Michael Lennington, which I absolutely endorse for anyone who would like to improve their life in a multitude of ways.

The fitness program set out in the pages below targets the initial 12 weeks of revitalizing exercises which form part of the overarching objective which you yourself will have constructed in your own mind. By the time the 12 weeks are up you will be well on your way to achieving what you have set out to achieve, and it will all seem so much easier.

You really need to exercise in some shape or form every day, almost without exception. Even though the main exercise routines normally take just 15 - 20 minutes, this will probably also require you to adjust your lifestyle in some way to accommodate them.

You will need to make a commitment. This becomes much easier if you reaffirm this daily, your commitment to achieve your goal.

You may have feelings of self-doubt from time to time, especially in the early days. In fact you probably will. It's at those times when you think that you are making little or no progress, that it is all too much effort, when you may need support. You could get support from someone who knows what it is like - me, for example - but the self-reinforcing belief that you **will** do what you set out to do comes from that little voice inside, when you revisit your objective that you defined and wrote down earlier.

Easy Fitness **is** easy, it really is. The only time when you may think that it is not easy at all is when you are first starting out, when you are unfamiliar with the exercises and your body starts to protest. Remember, your body is protesting for the very reason that these exercises are worth doing, for the very reason that some of your muscles have become unfamiliar with exercise. Unless your body is telling you that something is wrong, which is a very different thing. You should be able to recognize this difference, when you feel as though you will be causing yourself an injury if you continue.

What you need to remember is that you *will* become fit, you *will* have the improved body shape that you have set out to achieve. You just need to let yourself achieve it and continue with this program until you do. I will give you all the tools you need to get there, but only you can follow through with them. Your own personal determination will self-determine your results.

Just imagine. When you reach the plateau of easy fitness, what I call the maintenance level, it all becomes so easy that you will probably want to do more, just to challenge yourself.

# *Your Challenge*

Your first challenge, however, is to complete the first twelve weeks of this exercise program. The best way to do this is to set yourself a challenging target which will stretch you, and will mark a significant step towards your end goal. For example, if your end goal is to lose 50 pounds, your twelve week target could be to lose 20 pounds. If your end goal is to be fit enough to climb a 5,000ft mountain, your 12 week target could be to walk to the summit of a 1,000ft hill.

After doing this you should set yourself individual mini challenges for each of the next 12 weeks, separate from the exercises themselves. The exercises which I will be describing later are enough in themselves, of course, but other types of activity will broaden your fitness level and can significantly speed up your progress.

So first of all, set out your 12 Week Challenge here:

*My 12-Week Challenge is*..................................................................................................................

..................................................................................................................

**My Weekly Targets**
Make each one an *action* statement
e.g.
*By the end of this week –*
I will have walked 30 miles
I will have eaten only fresh food this week, no junk food
I will have refrained from any alcohol for the entire 7 days

I will have swum 10 lengths of the pool every day

By positioning these targets as accomplishments that you will have achieved, you are implying a commitment to yourself that these targets are ready and waiting to be ticked off, not merely a vague future promise to yourself.

Add as many as you like:

*By the end of this week –*

| I will... |
|---|
| I will... |
| I will... |
| I will... |
| I will... |
| I will... |
| I will... |

At the end of each week, tick off the successful accomplishment of each target. If you have missed any, score yourself out of 7 days, so that any day missed will count as 6/7. Try to make this the minimum score every week.

You will, of course, be feeling fitter as you progress through this first twelve weeks, so as the weeks go by you may wish to raise or lower your weekly targets. If you have been meeting them with ease then it's only fair to raise them a little, isn't it! It is best to wait until 4 weeks have been completed and then review the situation, and then do so again 4 weeks later. By that stage you will be amazed at how much fitter you are feeling, and what may have seemed challenging at first will pale into insignificance.

# THE THIRD STEP: GETTING READY FOR ACTION

At last we have reached the time to put words into action. Before you start, however, it is worth considering what equipment will help you.

## Equipment

One of the things I always emphasize about the **Easy Fitness** program is that no equipment is strictly necessary. There are certain items, though, which will make things even easier for you, but this is entirely for your own convenience. One thing is for sure, you definitely won't be needing any costly gym membership.

Here is what I use, purely by choice:

An **Exercise Mat**

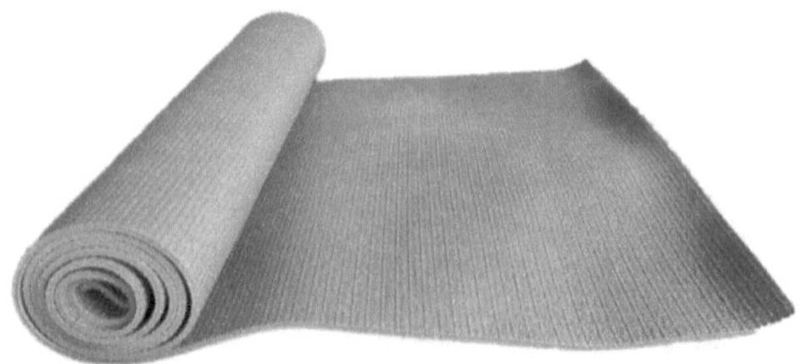

Also known as a yoga mat, such as the one shown above, this will help a lot unless you have beautifully cushioned flooring. Any discomfort you experience is best limited to pushing yourself harder to complete the exercises effectively.

## A **Pedometer**

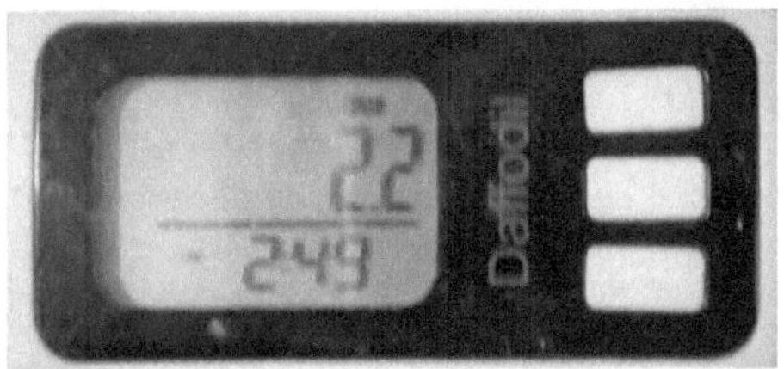

I recommend walking at least 12,000 steps a day, and although there are many smartphone apps which will count these for you, I find that a small pedometer such as the one shown above is better. You can carry this with you wherever you go and it is amazing how the steps rack up, even just moving around the home or office. I regularly find myself walking 16,000 steps without any real effort, just by being active and not taking short journeys by car.

You don't actually need a pedometer if you have a regular walk that lasts 30 minutes in each direction. Add this to an active day of walking to and fro around your local environment and this should add up to at least 12,000 steps. However, having a specific target which you can reach on a pedometer or smartphone app is much more satisfying, and will also drive you on to accomplish a few more steps when you would prefer just to put your feet up. Goals are a great motivator.

An alternative to the pedometer shown above would be a fitbit-style bracelet, which will track your movements throughout the day. You will really see the steps clock up from the moment you rise until the time you go to bed, and comparing this with a reading of the calories burned is another great motivator. The one shown here is good enough to measure steps, distance and calories, as well as waking you up 15–20 minutes earlier so that you can fit the *Easy Fitness* exercises into your busy schedule!

An actual fitbit 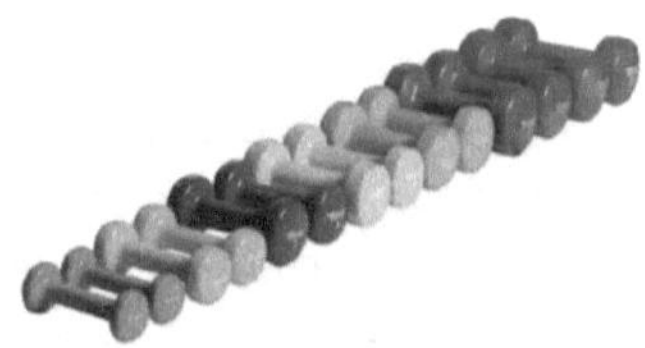 would probably be better, of course, but as with most of the 'equipment' described here, it is not strictly necessary.

**Walking Shoes**

It is important if you are stepping up your walking distances to 12,000 steps or more a day that you have a comfortable pair of shoes. There is no need to wear jogging or running shoes, but you should have footwear fit for the purpose when you become a frequent walker.

**Dumb Bells**, such as these York Barbells:

There is no weight-lifting involved in any of the exercises, but one particular exercise is great for toning the arms and flexing the chest. It is preferable to use a pair of dumb bells weighing 2kg (4 – 5 pounds) or more, depending on your size, though in the past I have used saucepans and they work just as well, as long as you take care to avoid overhead light bulbs!

## Let's Get Down to It

You are going to be pleasantly surprised as I reveal the exercises involved. Despite my emphasis on commitment, with a capital C, you will find that there isn't an incredibly daunting set of routines to match up to. Yes, it might be challenging at first for anyone who has not carried out any significant physical exercise for some time, but the program is deliberately structured so that you will gradually increase the exercise frequency from a fairly low base.

Your main commitment is to complete the course for the full 12 weeks (and then beyond) and achieve the aim you strongly desire. You will feel incredibly fulfilled, energized and much, much fitter at the end of this first 12 weeks, yet the exercise routines themselves should only take you around 15-20 minutes every day.

'Every Day' are two key words that are at the heart of this program. Sure, you will have a regular rest day for *active recovery*, but you will find that the daily exercises soon become an automatic part of your daily routine. Initially you will have to make time in your day for it, but ultimately it becomes a habit which seamlessly slots into your day.

You will soon discover how easy this all is. However, before we turn to the exercise schedule, I must first introduce another key element of this fitness plan.

# THE FOURTH STEP: IMPROVING YOUR DIET

The word diet is just a four-letter word, and yet many people may feel like using a four-letter word to describe a diet they have tried. In my opinion a lot of diets - in the form of diet***ing*** - are fools' gold. Yes, many diets work, and you may lose pound after pound while sticking to the regime, but how many of them are truly sustainable? If you can follow a particular diet for the rest of your life, and enjoy it, then good for you. For most people, dieting is a temporary measure and in the end reversion to the mean occurs. It seems almost as though you had never made the effort.

This course is not about dieting, nor even about weight loss, but losing excess weight will be a natural consequence of the exercises. Although after a while any weight loss may stabilize as you build more muscle, this initial weight loss should be permanent once you become fitter and lead a more active life.

When I use the term diet, I am referring to a **healthy** diet that reinforces the advances you have taken through exercise. Dieting does not come into it, and I always stress that there is no need to give up your favorite foods, as long as your overall food intake is based on a healthy, nutritious diet. I am a strong adherent of the Mediterranean diet as a foundation of many of my meals. This diet has been proven to be one of the healthiest in the world, and includes plenty of fresh vegetables and fruit, along with less use of red meats and foods lacking in genuine nutrition. You know which ones they are!

It's not rocket science. Observe the countries in the world whose citizens have a longer lifespan and think about what foods they eat. Although a healthy longevity may not entirely be down to a nation's diet, it does play a leading role.

With that in mind, here are some examples of the types of food which you should include in your diet as often as possible. They aren't necessarily low in calories, but they are recognized as nutritious *'superfoods'* which pass on many health benefits. By incorporating many of them into your regular eating patterns you will be laying the foundations for a healthier life.

> Aduki bean
> Alfalfa
> Almond
> Apple
> Apricot
> Asparagus
> Aubergine
> Avocado
> Banana
> Barley
> Beef (organic), in moderation
> Beetroot
> Bio-Yogurt
> Blueberry
> Brazil nut
> Broccoli
> Brussels Sprout
> Buckwheat
> Cabbage
> Camomile
> Canteloupe Melon
> Carrot
> Cashew nut
> Cauliflower
> Cayenne pepper
> Celery
> Cherry
> Chicken
> Chickpea
> Chilli pepper
> Cider Vinegar
> Cinnamon
> Coconut/Coconut oil
> Cranberry
> Cucumber
> Cumin
> Duck (skinned)

- Egg
- Fennel
- Fig
- Flaxseed
- Garlic
- Ginger
- Globe Artichoke
- Grape
- Grapefruit
- Green tea
- Honey
- Kale
- Kidney bean
- Kiwi Fruit
- Lamb
- Lemon
- Lentil
- Lettuce
- Mango
- Millet
- Mint
- Mushroom
- Oats
- Okra
- Olive/Olive Oil
- Onion
- Orange
- Oyster
- Papaya
- Parsley
- Pear
- Pepper
- Peppermint
- Pine nut
- Pineapple
- Plum/Prune
- Pomegranate
- Prawn
- Pumpkin seed
- Quinoa

- ➢ Raspberry
- ➢ Rice, brown
- ➢ Rosemary
- ➢ Rye
- ➢ Sage
- ➢ Salmon
- ➢ Sardine
- ➢ Seaweed
- ➢ Sesame seed/Sesame oil/Tahini
- ➢ Soya bean
- ➢ Spinach
- ➢ Squash
- ➢ Strawberry
- ➢ Sunflower seed/Sunflower oil
- ➢ Sweet Potato
- ➢ Tofu
- ➢ Tomato
- ➢ Tuna
- ➢ Turkey
- ➢ Turmeric
- ➢ Walnut
- ➢ Watercress
- ➢ Wheat/wheatgerm
- ➢ Yam
- ➢ Yogurt

If you include many of these superfoods in your diet regularly, they will go a long way towards protecting you from a variety of health issues which may come in later life, although they should not be seen as a cure-all for pre-existing conditions. Nor should they be eaten to excess - even superfoods should be eaten in moderation as part of a well-balanced diet.

## *Calories and Diet*

As we grow older, our bodies require fewer calories. Your metabolic rate slows with age, your body 'burning' calories at a reduced pace. This means that if you continue consuming the same quantities as you did during your 20s and 30s you will start to put on weight. Unless you exercise. You could cut down on your food consumption instead, but do you really want to do that? Unless you are already eating far too much, that is!

Your slowing metabolism will become increasingly apparent as you move into your fifties and sixties, but you are lucky enough to have bought this book so that you can take action now! Trust me, it will be much more difficult to act later, when you are ten or twenty years older. You don't want to be fat and fifty.

You can start now by keeping an eye on your calorie intake, balancing the calories you consume with the energy you are using throughout the day. You don't need to do this every day, but it is a good idea to take occasional weekly 'snapshots' of your calorie balance. I would recommend doing this for the duration of this initial 12-week program, or at least for one week out of four, which will help you establish a trend.

First of all, keep a diary itemizing whatever you eat and drink, which will give you a rough idea of your daily intake. You can download a free Interactive Calorie Chart here (https://easyfitnessforlife.net/free-reports) which will help you. If you can keep to the recommended calorie level, while simultaneously increasing your fitness level, then you will see the improvements that will be gained from the next few pages of exercise routines even more quickly.

If you need to lose - or gain - weight, then simply adjusting your daily intake by 500 calories will equate to one pound of weight each week. It is quite easy to do, just by asking yourself 'do I really need that extra slice, that extra drink?' - or is it just a habit? By doing this, and adding increased exercise into the mix, you will be amazed by the results.

The benefits of keeping a calorie diary are not limited purely to your weight. It is very easy to overlook the quality of your diet until you monitor it and see the reality, written down and confronting you with a pointed finger of shame when you contemplate it at the end of the week. Good health isn't just a matter of exercise and calorie limitation, and there are few things more important in the long term than what you put in your mouth. Think about switching to fruit, nuts and seeds, rather than cakes or crisps; to smoothies rather than fizzy drinks or frothy coffee; to wholegrain cereal and yoghurt as an alternative to pastries or fried foods.

# Nine Tips for a Healthy Diet

You can improve and maintain your future health by following these guidelines:

1. Drink plenty of water – at least six glasses a day. Avoid sugary drinks as much as possible, including those tempting coffees which are often packed with more sugar than you would believe!

2. Try to eat lower fat meat and dairy produce, and incorporate some alternatives into your diet, such as lentils, peas and eggs.

3. Fish - particularly the oily varieties such as mackerel, salmon, sardines, and tuna - would be a huge benefit for your weekly diet.

4. Drink less alcohol, making a point of considering whether you really do want another one. I know it can be easy to keep on topping up!

5. Eat a minimum of five portions of fruit and vegetables every day.

6. Eat a wide selection of foods, to gain a good balance of nutrients.

7. Steer clear of food and drinks with a high sugar or salt content, and avoid eating an excess of foods high in saturated fats. These include processed meats, fatty meats and chicken skin, as well as dairy products. Eat cheese and butter by all means, but keep an eye on the amounts, and try to have less in general. You can often use healthier substitutes, such as olive oil for cooking.

8. Check out labels. Keep an eye on the salt and sugar content, which may surprise you. Although these are visible on labels they are almost hidden in plain sight, because the amount of calories may be many people's first consideration. As a general rule, cutting back salt to less than 6 grams a day and avoiding any added sugars will benefit your health in the long run. Natural sugars in food are much more beneficial than added sugars.

9. Foods with starch possess the double benefits of being very low in fat, while also containing essential nutrients such as proteins, vitamins and minerals, along with essential fats. Include a good amount of starchy foods such as potatoes and sweet potatoes, wholegrain rice and breads, as well as breakfast cereals with oats and little or no added sugar.

For a much fuller explanation of healthy foods, you can also download this free e-book of *Simple Healthy Recipes* here (https://easyfitnessforlife.net/free-reports).

**The link between Exercise, Diet and Health**

By incorporating as many of these Nine Tips as you can into a well-balanced diet, while maintaining the recommended average calorie level and also following the exercises laid out in this program, you will be placing yourself firmly on the path towards a long and healthy life. In fact just by walking on a regular basis, as specified within the program, you can reduce your rate of physical decline by as much as 50%, which is quite an amazing figure.

# THE FIFTH STEP: EXERCISE STARTS HERE

Before you begin, it is vital that you take account of your existing fitness level. You should definitely consult your physician if you have done no exercise at all for months. If you are among the 40% of adults who don't even manage one brisk 10 minute walk a month, then just by beginning the walking aspects of this program you will be making a good start. However, any form of strenuous exercise is not recommended for anyone who has not exercised for many months or is clinically obese, without having first taken medical advice.

Even though the exercises which follow are not really difficult to complete, they may seem challenging at first because many of them may be unfamiliar to you, and to your unexercised body. For this reason they are graduated from a low level, which should be achievable for all but the medically unsound.

All of them are designed to be low impact in nature, but I must stress that if you are significantly overweight, have a history of health problems, or have undertaken little or no exercise for many months, then you should definitely start off at an even lower level than recommended below. Once again, I emphasize that medical advice should first be taken if you fall into any of those categories.

Explain the workout routines to your physician, and make it clear that this program is a graduated approach to greater fitness, designed for an average person in their forties. No account has been taken of any pre-existing medical conditions that you and your doctor will be aware of.

In any event, I can accept no responsibility for any injuries sustained while attempting any of the exercises or activities described, and you should be aware that it will always be a possibility that you may injure yourself while undertaking any form of physical activity.

Having said all that, these disclaimers should not contradict the fact that exercise is good for you. Nevertheless, you should start at a level which suits you. Everyone is different, and the following exercises are designed for a person with a reasonable fitness level who wishes to make a positive change to their life and their future prospects. If you are able to walk at a steady pace of 2.5 - 3mph (4 - 5kph) or more for at least 20 minutes, and without any known physical impediments, then you should be able to complete the first routines without difficulty. If you doubt that your fitness level is up to that standard, then I recommend that you start at a reduced level than set out in the course. I would suggest halving the amounts for the first two or three weeks, then aim to steadily catch up with the recommended levels within two months.

# Good Timing

Setting aside a specific twenty-minute time slot every day can certainly make it much easier to stick with the program. I personally prefer to exercise shortly after getting up in the morning, before breakfast. I get dressed into my exercise outfit, drink a glass or two of water to rehydrate myself, and keep a full glass within reach during my exercise routine. Less than twenty minutes later I am all set to start my day, refreshed, invigorated, and feeling very much the better for it.

One distinct advantage of exercising early in your day is the flow of positive energy which propels you through the morning. Besides feeling virtuous for the effort you have already put in before the day has truly got under way, you will also be experiencing the dopamine high which results from exercise. Dopamine is a neurotransmitter, stimulated by the endorphins activated by intensive exercise. Of course, as you know, the exercises set out in this book are termed 'easy', not 'intense', making it is unlikely that you would feel the full rush of this 'runner's high'. Nevertheless, a positive start to the day always feels good.

You may be unable to begin your day in this way, so by all means adapt your schedule to include twenty minutes of exercising at any time that suits you better. There is a risk that you may then have many reasons to keep putting it off, so I recommend that you ensure that there will be no distractions during any time slot which you allocate.

The third option, which you could consider as a last resort, is to fit in various exercises at odd moments throughout the day. This is perfectly possible to do, while waiting for the kettle to boil for example, as each element should only take two minutes or less. However, to reap the full benefits it is far preferable to complete the entire routine at the same time every day. It will then become a habit, to the point where it ceases being a chore to have to perform them, and becomes a fundamental part of your day, forming a virtuous circle.

# The Exercise Routines

The following sets of exercises should take you no more than 15 or 20 minutes every day. If you find that the routines are taking significantly longer than this, then you are probably performing the exercises too slowly or with too much commitment to perfection. Of course you should aim to complete each one to the best of your ability, but bear in mind that your ability will quickly improve with practice and familiarity. As you loosen up and become used to the exercises, you will find that within one week it will be possible to complete each exercise more quickly, more competently and more efficiently. In fact you will look back at your 'less fit' self just one week earlier and find it hard to imagine how you found any part of the routine difficult at all!

Wear loose clothing, such as a T-shirt or vest and shorts or tracksuit bottoms. I prefer to use a Yoga Mat for most of the exercises, as mentioned earlier.

Remind yourself of your grand vision, your entire reason for wanting to become fitter, and get ready to launch into:

# *WEEK ONE*

**DAY ONE**

Today is the day when you take control of your future fitness. Try as hard as you can, but don't push yourself excessively at this early stage. Be prepared for a longer session than will become usual, as you will be familiarising yourself with the exercises for the first time.

### *Limbering Up*

**Toe Touches**

i)      Stand with your feet flat to the floor, approximately one foot (30cm) apart.

ii)     Gently rise onto your toes, stretching both arms upwards as far as you can reach towards the ceiling, sucking your stomach in.

iii)    Feet flat on the floor once again, bend forwards to touch your toes, or the floor if you can manage it.

iv)    Straighten up and repeat.

Begin with 10 in total

*Excellent exercise for the calves, bottom, upper & lower back, and arms*

**Arm Rotations**

i)      Raise both arms and rotate them forwards in a circular motion

ii)     Repeat 4 more times

iii)    Reverse the direction to complete a backwards circular motion

iv)    Repeat 4 more times

*Improves flexibility, tones the chest and upper back*

**Lateral Body Bends**

i)      Stand with your feet approximately 18 inches (45 cm) apart, placing both hands behind your head.

ii)     Hold your stomach in, and then bend your body sideways from the waist as far as it feels comfortable to do so. Preferably you will achieve something approaching a 45 degree angle, but you should at least feel your muscles pulling from the waist at the side, which is as it should be if you want to make a difference to your waistline.

iii)    Return to the center and repeat to the opposite side.

iv)    Repeat with 9 more bends to each side

*Strengthens the spine, tones your waist and torso muscles, will help eradicate flab!*

**Alternate Toe Touches**

i)      Stand with your feet flat to the floor, approximately one foot apart.

ii)     Swing your left arm in a circular motion over your head and bend down toward the right until your hand reaches the little toe of your right foot.

iii)    Straighten up, and then repeat with the right arm reaching down to your left foot.

iv)     Repeat this movement 4 more times on each side

*For a trim waist, toned thighs, and a supple lower back*

**Running On The Spot**

Jog up and down gently, lifting your legs three to four inches (7 – 10 cm) from the floor and coming down softly on your toes, for a period of 30 seconds (or count to 30 slowly).

*Tones your hips and thighs, and raises your heart rate*

## *Core Training*

**Abdominal Strength Training**

i)      Lie on your back, arms to the side, knees bent at 35-40 degrees, with your feet flat on the floor.

ii)     Suck your stomach in, while raising your head and shoulders off the floor.

iii)    Hold this position, continuing to hold your stomach in as much as possible, while also raising your legs off the floor, knees bent with the lower leg straight so that you can see your toes. Hold this position for a count of 5.

iv)     Lower your legs, still bent, with a controlled motion, feeling the pull on your stomach as you do so.

v)      As you lower your legs relax your head and shoulders back to the floor.

vi)     Repeat four more times

*This isometric exercise is wonderful for the waistline, pulling on the lower abdominal muscles for a firm, toned stomach*

**Laid Back Kicks**

i)      Sit on the floor, leaning backwards with your knees bent, supporting your upper body with your hands on the floor behind you.

ii)     Raise one leg 30-40 cm (12 – 16 inches) above the floor, knee still bent, and then stretch out in a kicking motion.

iii)    As you do so, raise the other leg, knee bent, and kick out with this leg as you retract the first leg to a raised, knee bent, position.

iv)     Repeat this alternate kicking motion until you have kicked 15 times with each leg.

*Tightens the abdomen and tones the thighs*

## Thigh Squeezes

i)      Stand with both legs approximately 18 inches (45 cm) apart, hands on your hips.

ii)     Tighten your thigh muscles firmly, pushing your feet hard into the floor, for a count of 5. You will feel your abdomen tightening as you do so.

iii)    Repeat this twice more for a total of 3 thigh squeezes.

iv)     Next, widen your stance, so that your legs are approximately 24 inches (60 cm) apart, and then repeat the squeezes 3 more times, each with a count of 5.

v)      Continue to widen your legs by approximately 6 inches (15 cm) each time, squeezing 3 times on each occasion, until you are unable to maintain the position comfortably. Repeat 5 more times

*Tones and strengthens the thighs, and will work wonders for your walking speed*

## Lateral Leg Raises

i)      Lie down on your right side, arms to the side, both legs together.

ii)     Raise your left leg high into the air, as high as you can, forming a V shape.

iii)    Lower your leg slowly, controlling the descent with your thigh muscles.

iv)     Repeat 14 more times, then turn onto your left side and repeat the process.

*Excellent exercise for the leg muscles, also your hips and waist*

***Cool Down***

## Lateral Leans

i)      Stand up straight, legs about 1 foot (30cm) apart, suck your stomach in then bend your body to the side, reaching towards the knee.

ii)     Straighten up again, and repeat the process to the other side.

iii)    Repeat 9 more times

*Feel that pull on your waist as you stretch to each side. Another flab eliminator*

**Forward Bend & Stretch**

N.B.  This exercise will improve blood flow to the brain over time. However, you should stop immediately if you feel at all dizzy.

i)      Stand with your feet approximately 9 - 12 inches (23 - 30 cm) apart, knees slightly bent.

ii)     Lower your chin towards the collar bone, and gently roll your body forwards from the waist, arms hanging to the front, until your fingers are hanging just above your feet.

iii)    Maintaining this loose, dangling posture, chin still held in a downwards position, pull your stomach back towards the base of your spine while breathing in slowly and deeply for a count of 3, and then exhale slowly.

iv)     Repeat this twice more.

v)      Now slowly unroll your body to a standing position, and imagine that your back is rolling up against a wall.

vi)     When you are at your full height, chin still lowered, continue the rolling back motion to arch your back a little and raise both arms above your head.

vii)    Now repeat the earlier abdominal exercise, breathing in deeply three times for a count of 3.

viii)   Finally, relax and bring both arms down to your side in a flowing circular motion.

ix)     Raise your chin and rotate your neck from side to side and up and down.

x)      Repeat this exercise 2 more times.

*Relaxing, and terrific for your waistline, pulling on the lower abdominal muscles for a firmer stomach, while also strengthening your spine and legs*

This completes your exercise routine for the day, and will probably have taken longer than 20 minutes. Don't despair – you <u>will</u> speed up!

Walk up and down for approximately 30 seconds as your pulse rate reduces.

**Daily Steps:** 10,000 minimum (approximately 3 miles)

**DAY TWO**

Your body is quite possibly feeling a little stiff after the unfamiliar exercises yesterday. This is normal, and unless you are feeling any undue pain, proceed gently with your second day. Believe me, you will loosen up soon after beginning, and it will all become easier over time. Starting is difficult, finishing is easy.

### *Limbering Up*

**Toe Touches** - 10
**Arm Rotations** - 5 forwards, 5 backwards
**Lateral Body Bends** - 10 to each side
**Alternate Toe Touches** - 5 to each side
**Running On The Spot** - 30 seconds

### *Core Training*

**Abdominal Strength Training** - 5
**Laid Back Kicks** - 15 with each leg
**Thigh Squeezes** - 6 sets
**Lateral Leg Raises** - 15 on each side

### *Cool Down*

**Lateral Leans** - 10 each side
**Forward Bend & Stretch** - 3

Walk up and down for approximately 30 seconds as your pulse rate reduces.

**Daily Steps:** 10,000 minimum (approximately 3 miles)

**DAY THREE**

### *Limbering Up*

**Toe Touches** - 11
**Arm Rotations** - 6 forwards, 6 backwards
**Lateral Body Bends** - 11 to each side
**Alternate Toe Touches** - 6 to each side
**Running On The Spot** - 35 seconds

### *Core Training*

**Leg-Passing Knee Pulls**

i)    Lie on your back, arms to the side, knees bent, heels resting on the floor.

ii)   Raise one leg, and bring it up close to your chest, pulling the knee firmly down with clasped hands. Hold this position for a count of 5.

iii)  As you return this leg to its starting position, repeat the movement with your other leg, so that both legs pass in mid-air.

iv)   Repeat these alternating knee pulls 4 more times with each leg, until 5 sequences have been completed.

*Excellent exercise for the thighs, bottom and hips*


**Abdominal Strength Training - 6**
**Thigh Squeezes - 7 sets**


**Ab Lifts**

N.B.   I recommend that all exercises in the *Easy Fitness For Over 40s* plan are best done in the morning before breakfast, but it is particularly true with this exercise, preferably with an empty stomach. Also, please note that if you currently have, or have had abdominal issues in the past, you should refer to your doctor before undertaking this powerful exercise.

i)    Stand with your feet approximately 9 - 12 inches (23 - 30 cm) apart

ii)   Bend forwards gently and rest your hands just above each knee

iii)  Breathe out forcefully, emptying your lungs

iv)   Without breathing in, pull your abdomen strongly inwards, as though you are trying to pull it back to your spine, then hold this for 5-10 seconds

v)    Breathe in gently a couple of times

vi)   Repeat from step iii), and then do so once more, making 3 in total

vii)  Now stand back upright again, arms loosely by the side, then raise both arms in front of you, continuing to raise them until they are high above your head, stretching up as far as you comfortably can

viii) Next hold your breath for about 5 seconds, feeling your abs stretch taut as you do so, then breathe in once more.

ix)   Repeat steps ii) – viii) three times more


*This traditional Chinese exercise is very similar to Indian yoga, and counteracts abdominal sag, as well as strengthening your diaphragm. This will aid your breathing -*

*particularly useful for fitness exercises in general - and is also beneficial for and preventative of digestive problems*

### *Cool Down*

**Lateral Leans** - 11 each side
**Forward Bend & Stretch** - 3

Walk up and down for approximately 30 seconds as your pulse rate reduces.

**Daily Steps:** 10,000 minimum (approximately 3 miles)

## DAY FOUR

### *Limbering Up Only*

**Toe Touches** - 11
**Arm Rotations** - 6 forwards, 6 backwards
**Lateral Body Bends** - 11 to each side
**Alternate Toe Touches** - 6 to each side
**Running On The Spot** - 35 seconds

## DAY FIVE

### *Limbering Up*

**Toe Touches** - 12
**Arm Rotations** - 7 forwards, 7 backwards
**Lateral Body Bends** - 12 to each side
**Alternate Toe Touches** - 7 to each side
**Running On The Spot** - 40 seconds

### *Core Training*

**Leg-Passing Knee Pulls** - 5
**Abdominal Strength Training** - 6
**Thigh Squeezes** - 7 sets
**Ab Lifts** - 4

### *Cool Down*

**Lateral Leans** - 11 each side
**Forward Bend & Stretch** - 3

Walk up and down for approximately 30 seconds as your pulse rate reduces.

**Daily Steps:** 10,000 minimum (approximately 3 miles)

**DAY SIX**

### *Limbering Up*

**Toe Touches** - 12
**Arm Rotations** - 7 forwards, 7 backwards
**Lateral Body Bends** - 12 to each side
**Alternate Toe Touches** - 7 to each side
**Running On The Spot** - 40 seconds

### *Core Training*

**Abdominal Strength Training** - 7
**Laid Back Kicks** - 16 with each leg
**Thigh Squeezes** - 8 sets
**Lateral Leg Raises** - 16 on each side

### *Cool Down*

**Lateral Leans** - 12 each side
**Forward Bend & Stretch** - 3

Walk up and down for approximately 30 seconds as your pulse rate reduces.

**Daily Steps:** 10,000 minimum (approximately 3 miles)

**DAY SEVEN**

### *Limbering Up*

**Toe Touches** - 13
**Arm Rotations** - 8 forwards, 8 backwards
**Lateral Body Bends** - 13 to each side
**Alternate Toe Touches** - 8 to each side
**Running On The Spot** - 45 seconds

### *Core Training*

**Leg-Passing Knee Pulls** - 6
**Abdominal Strength Training** - 7
**Thigh Squeezes** - 8 sets
**Ab Lifts** - 5

### *Cool Down*

**Lateral Leans** - 12 each side
**Forward Bend & Stretch** - 3

Walk up and down for approximately 30 seconds as your pulse rate reduces.

**Daily Steps:** 10,000 minimum (approximately 3 miles)

So how is going so far? Tough going, or as easy as I promised? You should be noticing some early signs of real improvement very soon, probably over the next week. But only if you have completed **all** the exercises to the best of your ability, and also hit an 85% strike rate on your own Weekly Targets. You will already be loosening up nicely and, even though it is early days, you may just be starting to feel some of your clothes hanging differently on you.

# WEEK TWO

**DAY ONE**

### *Limbering Up*

**Toe Touches** - 13
**Arm Rotations** - 8 forwards, 8 backwards
**Lateral Body Bends** - 13 to each side
**Alternate Toe Touches** - 8 to each side
**Running On The Spot** - 45 seconds

### *Core Training*

**Reverse Curl Ups**

i)  Lie on the floor, arms to the side.
ii)  Pull both knees up to your chest so that your bottom is off the floor, and cross your ankles as your knees move upwards, keeping the knees wide apart.
iii)  Firmly hold your knees or shins close to your chest with both arms, as though hugging your legs, for a count of 5, then release and straighten your legs, lowering them to the floor in a controlled motion.
iv)  Repeat four times more.

*For a firmer bottom and thighs, also aids hip flexibility, and works your pelvic floor muscles together with your lower abdomen and lumbar area*

**Laid Back Kicks** - 16 with each leg

**Arm Lifts**

i)  Raise your right arm to the side, reaching high above the shoulder.
ii)  Repeat four times more, and then perform the same action with your left arm five times.
iii)  Now repeat, using both arms simultaneously, completing 5 lifts, to total 15 rounds in all.

After this gentle introduction to arm raises, it will be a great improvement to do this exercise using small weights. I personally use two small 2.5 kg (one pound, approx.) dumbbell-style weights (any size ranging between 1.5kg and 3kg will do, depending on your size). This is intended for arm-toning and shoulder strength, rather than gaining massive biceps, so it is not necessary to have weights which are heavier than you can comfortably carry.

There is no need to use weights which create a heavy pull on your arms as a heavy shopping bag would. If you prefer not to make the investment then you will be fine with any household object of roughly equivalent weight, as long as it is fairly small and easy to grip.

*Excellent exercise for flabby or un-toned upper arms, for shoulder strength, and a good waist stretcher*

### Head & Shoulder Lifts

i)      Lie on your back, legs straight, arms to the side.

ii)     Raise your head and both shoulders off the floor, while pulling your abdominal muscles gently downwards at the same time. Hold this position for a count of 5, and then relax, slowly lowering your head and shoulders back to the floor.

iii)    Repeat this exercise 9 more times.

*A gentle exercise which tightens the abdomen and strengthens the neck*

### *Cool Down*

**Lateral Leans** – 13 each side
**Forward Bend & Stretch**   4

Walk up and down for approximately 30 seconds as your pulse rate reduces.

**Daily Steps:** 10,000 minimum (approximately 3 miles)

### DAY TWO
Rest Day

### *Limbering Up Only*

**Toe Touches** – 14
**Arm Rotations** – 9 forwards, 9 backwards
**Lateral Body Bends** – 14 to each side
**Alternate Toe Touches** – 9 to each side
**Running On The Spot** – 50 seconds

**Daily Steps:** 10,000 minimum (approximately 3 miles)

**DAY THREE**

*Limbering Up*

**Toe Touches** - 14
**Arm Rotations** - 9 forwards, 9 backwards
**Lateral Body Bends** - 14 to each side
**Alternate Toe Touches** - 9 to each side
**Running On The Spot** - 50 seconds

*Core Training*

**Reverse Curl Ups** - 5
**Laid Back Kicks** - 17 with each leg
**Arm Lifts** – 15 (5 Left, 5 Right, 5 together)
**Head & Shoulder Lifts** - 10

*Cool Down*

**Lateral Leans** - 13 each side
**Forward Bend & Stretch** - 4

Walk up and down for approximately 30 seconds as your pulse rate reduces.

**Daily Steps:** 10,000 minimum (approximately 3 miles)

**DAY FOUR**

*Limbering Up*

**Toe Touches** - 15
**Arm Rotations** - 10 forwards, 10 backwards
**Lateral Body Bends** - 15 to each side
**Alternate Toe Touches** - 10 to each side
**Running On The Spot** - 55 seconds

*Core Training*

**Leg-Passing Knee Pulls** - 6

**Calf Stretches**

i)      Stand approximately 3 feet from a wall, or you could use a door frame

ii)     Lean forward so that both arms are stretched out against the wall (or door frame)

iii)    Step forward with your right foot, bending the knee, so that the toe is nearly touching the wall, keeping your left foot flat to the ground, leg straight, so that it is forming a 45% angle with the floor. Bend your right knee slightly, until you feel the calf muscle in your left leg stretching. If this feels uncomfortable then you are bending your knee too much. Hold this for a count of 5.

iv)     Now step back with the left foot, keeping it flat to the floor adjacent to your right foot, and step forward with your right leg, knee bent, so that the foot is close to the wall. Hold this for a count of 5.

v)      Repeat this exercise 6 more times with each leg.

*Good exercise for the calf muscles, will help you power up those hills*

**Lateral Leg Raises** - 16 on each side

**Stepped Push-ups (Male)**

i)      Lie face down on the floor, legs straight, both arms bent at the elbow, palm down, in the push-up position.

ii)     Now step your right arm and your right leg out wide, and push upwards, straightening your arms as you raise your body, then control your descent to the floor.

iii)    Repeat with the left arm and leg stepped out wide.

iv)     Repeat four more times.

Although this is a non-impact push-up, with less strain on your back and better shoulder movement, you may still find this exercise quite difficult at first if you have not done push-ups for a long time. If this is the case, you will find it easier to kneel than to have your legs fully extended, and continue with this version of the exercise until your arm strength has improved.

*Tones the upper arms to eradicate flabbiness, as well as being excellent exercise for the shoulders and chest*

**Diamond Push-ups (Female only)**

i)      Lie face down on the floor, arms to the side.

ii)     Move your hands together below the breastbone, forming a triangle shape with your thumb and forefingers.

iii)      Push upwards to straighten your arms at the elbow.

iv)      Repeat four more times

*Tones the upper arms, counteracting arm 'jiggle', as well as being excellent exercise for the shoulders and chest*

### *Cool Down*

**Lateral Leans** - 14 each side
**Forward Bend & Stretch** - 4

Walk up and down for approximately 30 seconds as your pulse rate reduces.

**Daily Steps:** 10,000 minimum (approximately 3 miles)

**DAY FIVE**

### *Limbering Up*

**Toe Touches** - 15
**Arm Rotations** - 10 forwards, 10 backwards
**Lateral Body Bends** - 15 to each side
**Alternate Toe Touches** - 10 to each side
**Running On The Spot** - 55 seconds

### *Core Training*

**Leg-Passing Knee Pulls** - 7
**Calf Stretches** - 7
**Lateral Leg Raises** - 17 on each side
**Stepped Push Ups (male)** - 5
**Diamond Push Ups (female)** - 5

### *Cool Down*

**Lateral Leans** - 14 each side
**Forward Bend & Stretch** - 4

Walk up and down for approximately 30 seconds as your pulse rate reduces.

**Daily Steps:** 10,000 minimum (approximately 3 miles)

**DAY SIX**

### *Limbering Up*

**Toe Touches** - 16
**Arm Rotations** - 11 forwards, 11 backwards
**Lateral Body Bends** - 16 to each side
**Alternate Toe Touches** - 10 to each side
**Running On The Spot** - 60 seconds

### *Core Training*

**Reverse Curl Ups** - 6
**Laid Back Kicks** - 17 with each leg
**Arm Lifts** - 16 (5 Left, 5 Right, 6 together)
**Head & Shoulder Lifts** - 11

### *Cool Down*

**Lateral Leans** - 15 each side
**Forward Bend & Stretch** - 4

Walk up and down for approximately 30 seconds as your pulse rate reduces.

**Daily Steps:** 10,000 minimum (approximately 3 miles)

**DAY SEVEN**

### *Limbering Up*

**Toe Touches** - 16
**Arm Rotations** - 11 forwards, 11 backwards
**Lateral Body Bends** - 16 to each side
**Alternate Toe Touches** - 10 to each side
**Running On The Spot** - 60 seconds

### *Core Training*

**Leg-Passing Knee Pulls** - 7
**Calf Stretches** - 8
**Lateral Leg Raises** - 17 on each side
**Stepped Push Ups (male)** - 6
**Diamond Push Ups (female)** - 6

*Cool Down*

**Lateral Leans** - 15 each side
**Forward Bend & Stretch** - 4

Walk up and down for approximately 30 seconds as your pulse rate reduces.

**Daily Steps:** 10,000 minimum (approximately 3 miles)

Now we are really making progress...

# WEEK THREE

**DAY ONE**

*Limbering Up*

**Toe Touches** - 17
**Arm Rotations** - 12 forwards, 12 backwards
**Lateral Body Bends** - 17 to each side
**Alternate Toe Touches** - 10 to each side
**Running On The Spot** - 65 seconds

*Core Training*

**Abdominal Strength Training** - 8

**Roll Backs**
i)       Lie on your back on the floor, arms to the side.
ii)      Raise both legs, keeping them together, and stretch them back as far as
         is comfortable over your head. The aim is for your toes to touch the floor

behind you, but that is not possible for everyone. Try your hardest to get as close to the floor as you can. If your feet are still several inches or centimetres from the floor your effort will be equally beneficial.

iii)  As you reverse the position try to control the descent as you lower your legs to the floor, and resist the opposing force that will pull your shoulders off the floor. You should feel your lower abdomen stretching as your legs near the ground. Repeat four more times.

*Good exercise to enhance the abdomen, tone thigh muscles and strengthen the lower back*

**Arm Lifts** - 16
**Thigh Squeezes** - 9 sets

### *Cool Down*

**Lateral Leans** - 16 each side
**Forward Bend & Stretch** - 5

Walk up and down for approximately 30 seconds as your pulse rate reduces.

**Daily Steps:** 10,000 minimum (approximately 3 miles)

**DAY TWO**

### *Limbering Up Only*

**Toe Touches** - 17
**Arm Rotations** - 12 forwards, 12 backwards
**Lateral Body Bends** - 17 to each side
**Alternate Toe Touches** - 10 to each side
**Running On The Spot** - 65 seconds

**Daily Steps:** 10,000 minimum (approximately 3 miles)

**DAY THREE**

### *Limbering Up*

**Toe Touches** - 18
**Arm Rotations** - 13 forwards, 13 backwards
**Lateral Body Bends** - 18 to each side

**Alternate Toe Touches** - 10 to each side
**Running On The Spot** - 70 seconds

### *Core Training*

**Abdominal Strength Training** - 8
**Roll Backs** - 5
**Arm Lifts** - 17 (5 Left, 5 Right, 7 together)
**Thigh Squeezes** - 9 sets

### *Cool Down*

**Lateral Leans** - 16 each side
**Forward Bend & Stretch** - 5

Walk up and down for approximately 30 seconds as your pulse rate reduces.

**Daily Steps:** 10,000 minimum (approximately 3 miles)

**DAY FOUR**

### *Limbering Up*

**Toe Touches** - 18
**Arm Rotations** - 13 forwards, 13 backwards
**Lateral Body Bends** - 18 to each side
**Alternate Toe Touches** - 10 to each side
**Running On The Spot** - 70 seconds

### *Core Training*

**Calf Stretches** - 8
**Hand and Foot**
This exercise requires more space than most, at least three feet on either side of you.

    i)        Lie flat on the floor, arms by the side
    ii)       Stretch your left arm out at a right angle, palm flat to the floor
    iii)     Now swing your right leg over your body, keeping it stiff, and try to touch the tips of the fingers of your left hand with the toes of your right

foot. Get as close as you can, even if your toes and fingers are not touching.

iv)       Return your right leg to your side, and repeat 9 more times.

v)        Now return the left arm to your side, and stretch out your right arm.

vi)       Raise your left leg and repeat (iii).

vii)      When you have repeated (vi) nine more times, return to position (i)

*An excellent strengthening exercise for the waist muscles, good also for firming and toning your thighs*

**Laid Back Kicks** - 18 with each leg
**Ab Lifts** - 5

### *Cool Down*

**Lateral Leans** - 17 each side
**Forward Bend & Stretch** - 5

Walk up and down for approximately 30 seconds as your pulse rate reduces.

**Daily Steps:** 10,000 minimum (approximately 3 miles)

**DAY FIVE**

### *Limbering Up*

**Toe Touches** - 19
**Arm Rotations** - 14 forwards, 14 backwards
**Lateral Body Bends** - 19 to each side
**Alternate Toe Touches** - 10 to each side
**Running On The Spot** - 75 seconds

### *Core Training*

**Calf Stretches** - 9
**Hand and Foot** - 10
**Laid Back Kicks** - 18 with each leg
**Ab Lifts** - 6

### *Cool Down*

**Lateral Leans** - 17 each side
**Forward Bend & Stretch** - 5

Walk up and down for approximately 30 seconds as your pulse rate reduces.

**Daily Steps:** 10,000 minimum (approximately 3 miles)


**DAY SIX**

### *Limbering Up*

**Toe Touches** - 19
**Arm Rotations** - 14 forwards, 14 backwards
**Lateral Body Bends** - 19 to each side
**Alternate Toe Touches** - 10 to each side
**Running On The Spot** - 75 seconds

### *Core Training*

**Abdominal Strength Training** - 9
**Roll Backs** - 6
**Arm Lifts** - 17 (5 Left, 5 Right, 7 together)
**Thigh Squeezes** - 10 sets

### *Cool Down*

**Lateral Leans** - 18 each side
**Forward Bend & Stretch** - 5

Walk up and down for approximately 30 seconds as your pulse rate reduces.

**Daily Steps:** 10,000 minimum (approximately 3 miles)


**DAY SEVEN**

### *Limbering Up*

**Toe Touches** - 20
**Arm Rotations** - 15 forwards, 15 backwards
**Lateral Body Bends** - 20 to each side

**Alternate Toe Touches** – 10 to each side
**Running On The Spot** – 80 seconds

### *Core Training*

**Calf Stretches** – 9
**Hand and Foot** – 11
**Laid Back Kicks** – 19 with each leg
**Ab Lifts** – 6

### *Cool Down*

**Lateral Leans** – 18 each side
**Forward Bend & Stretch** – 5

Walk up and down for approximately 30 seconds as your pulse rate reduces.

**Daily Steps:** 10,000 minimum (approximately 3 miles)

# WEEK FOUR

**DAY ONE**

### *Limbering Up*

**Toe Touches** – 20
**Arm Rotations** – 15 forwards, 15 backwards
**Lateral Body Bends** – 20 to each side
**Alternate Toe Touches** – 10 to each side
**Running On The Spot** – 80 seconds

### *Core Training*

**Reverse Curl Ups** – 6
**Arm Lifts** – 18 (6 Left, 6 Right, 6 together)
**Head & Shoulder Lifts** – 11

**Full Sit Ups**

**N.B.** If you feel significant back pain while doing this exercise you should stop immediately

   i)      Lie down with your head resting on the floor, legs straight, arms across your chest with your hands resting on each shoulder.

   ii)     Tighten your stomach and raise your head and shoulders off the floor as far as you can.

   iii)    Keep your arms across your chest as you do so, and try as hard as you can to sit up and lean forward towards your toes.

This is a difficult – but ultimately very rewarding – exercise, and it is quite unlikely that you will be able to achieve this at your first attempt.

   iv)    Repeat this four more times, trying each time to sit up as far as you can. If all you can do at this stage is to raise your head and shoulders off the floor and little more than that, then this is exactly the position I found myself in several years ago. What will happen when you persevere is that suddenly you will amaze yourself and sit right up. Maybe this week, maybe on the next week for these exercises, maybe later – but it will happen. Hard to believe at first, but when you have done this once then you can continue to do it several more times, keeping up a good rhythm. Something to show off to your friends!

*When done properly, this is massively beneficial for your abdominal muscles, and will create a taut abdomen that you would never have believed possible*

### *Cool Down*

**Lateral Leans** - 19 each side
**Forward Bend & Stretch** - 5

**DAY TWO**

### *Limbering Up*

**Toe Touches** - 21
**Arm Rotations** - 16 forwards, 16 backwards
**Lateral Body Bends** - 20 to each side
**Alternate Toe Touches** - 10 to each side
**Running On The Spot** - 85 seconds

### *Core Training*

**Reverse Curl Ups** - 7
**Arm Lifts** - 18 (6 Left, 6 Right, 6 together)

**Head & Shoulder Lifts** - 12
**Full Sit Ups** - 5

### *Cool Down*

**Lateral Leans** - 19 each side
**Forward Bend & Stretch** - 5

Walk up and down for approximately 30 seconds as your pulse rate reduces.

**Daily Steps:** 10,000 minimum (approximately 3 miles)

## DAY THREE

### *Limbering Up Only*

**Toe Touches** - 21
**Arm Rotations** - 16 forwards, 16 backwards
**Lateral Body Bends** - 20 to each side
**Alternate Toe Touches** - 10 to each side
**Running On The Spot** - 85 seconds

**Daily Steps:** 10,000 minimum (approximately 3 miles)

## DAY FOUR

### *Limbering Up*

**Toe Touches** - 22
**Arm Rotations** - 17 forwards, 17 backwards
**Lateral Body Bends** - 20 to each side
**Alternate Toe Touches** - 10 to each side
**Running On The Spot** - 90 seconds

### *Core Training*

**Abdominal Strength Training** - 9
**Lateral Leg Raises** - 18 on each side
**Calf Stretches** - 10

**Pendulum Leg Swings**

You will need quite a lot of space around you for this one.

i)      Lie on the floor, arms to the side.

ii)     Keeping both legs together, lift them vertically into the air, then swing to the left in a controlled motion, stopping just before your feet touch the floor.

iii)    Now swing both legs back up and over to the right.

iv)     Repeat this four more times.

*You will immediately feel the 'pull' on your abdomen as your muscle stretches (to become better-toned over time), and this is also a great exercise for reducing any flab on your waist and hips.*

### *Cool Down*

**Lateral Leans** - 20 each side
**Forward Bend & Stretch** - 5

Walk up and down for approximately 30 seconds as your pulse rate reduces.

**Daily Steps:** 10,000 minimum (approximately 3 miles)

**DAY FIVE**

### *Limbering Up*

**Toe Touches** - 22
**Arm Rotations** - 17 forwards, 17 backwards
**Lateral Body Bends** - 20 to each side
**Alternate Toe Touches** - 10 to each side
**Running On The Spot** - 90 seconds

### *Core Training*

**Abdominal Strength Training** - 10
**Lateral Leg Raises** - 18 on each side
**Calf Stretches** - 10
**Pendulum Leg Swings** - 5

### *Cool Down*

**Lateral Leans** - 20 each side
**Forward Bend & Stretch** - 5

Walk up and down for approximately 30 seconds as your pulse rate reduces.

**Daily Steps:** 10,000 minimum (approximately 3 miles)


**DAY SIX**

*Limbering Up*

**Toe Touches** - 23
**Arm Rotations** - 18 forwards, 18 backwards
**Lateral Body Bends** - 20 to each side
**Alternate Toe Touches** - 10 to each side
**Running On The Spot** - 95 seconds

*Core Training*

**Reverse Curl Ups** - 7
**Arm Lifts** - 19 (6 Left, 6 Right, 7 together)
**Head & Shoulder Lifts** - 12
**Full Sit Ups** - 6

*Cool Down*

**Lateral Leans** - 20 each side
**Forward Bend & Stretch** - 5

Walk up and down for approximately 30 seconds as your pulse rate reduces.

**Daily Steps:** 10,000 minimum (approximately 3 miles)


**DAY SEVEN**

*Limbering Up*

**Toe Touches** - 23
**Arm Rotations** - 18 forwards, 18 backwards
**Lateral Body Bends** - 20 to each side

**Alternate Toe Touches** - 10 to each side
**Running On The Spot** - 95 seconds

### *Core Training*

**Abdominal Strength Training** - 10
**Lateral Leg Raises** - 19 on each side
**Calf Stretches** - 11
**Pendulum Leg Swings** - 6

### *Cool Down*

**Lateral Leans** - 20 each side
**Forward Bend & Stretch** - 5

Walk up and down for approximately 30 seconds as your pulse rate reduces.

**Daily Steps:** 10,000 minimum (approximately 3 miles)


Four Weeks completed. Congratulations on showing the determination to get this far. Now it is time to take stock and review your Weekly Targets which you set just over 4 weeks ago. Are you achieving an 85% strike rate (about 6 days out of 7, for example), or has it been a struggle? Now is the time to re-align yourself with your main vision, your overriding goal, and re-set your targets to make sure you get there. If you feel that you should set your targets a little lower then that is OK. It is difficult to set targets at exactly the right level until you get used to setting them. The same applies if you have found your targets not challenging enough (achieving 100% every week without any real effort, for example). Try again, and make it better this time. We are nearly ready to go again, into the fifth week and beyond!

How about the main Exercise Plan? You should be achieving at least an 85% strike rate, and preferably 100% if you are to gain the full benefits from this program. If you are achieving 100% completion then that is ideal. It will all become easier and easier for you to take on the exercises, even as they are increasing in number. You should also find that you can put more effort into them and be executing them more perfectly as every day goes by. As you grow fitter, what once seemed quite daunting becomes relatively insignificant.

# WEEK FIVE

**DAY ONE**

### *Limbering Up*

**Toe Touches** - 24
**Arm Rotations** - 19 forwards, 19 backwards
**Lateral Body Bends** - 20 to each side
**Alternate Toe Touches** - 10 to each side
**Running On The Spot** - 100 seconds

### *Core Training*

**Leg-Passing Knee Pulls** - 8
**Ab Lifts** - 7
**Stepped Push Ups (male)** - 6
**Diamond Push Ups (female)** - 6
**Thigh Squeezes** - 10 sets

### *Cool Down*

**Lateral Leans** - 20 each side
**Forward Bend & Stretch** - 5

Walk up and down for approximately 30 seconds as your pulse rate reduces.

**Daily Steps:** 10,000 minimum (approximately 3 miles)

**DAY TWO**

### *Limbering Up*

**Toe Touches** - 24
**Arm Rotations** - 19 forwards, 19 backwards
**Lateral Body Bends** - 20 to each side

**Alternate Toe Touches** - 10 to each side
**Running On The Spot** - 100 seconds

### *Core Training*

**Leg-Passing Knee Pulls** - 8
**Ab Lifts** - 7
**Stepped Push Ups (male)** - 7
**Diamond Push Ups (female)** - 7
**Thigh Squeezes** - 10 sets

### *Cool Down*

**Lateral Leans** - 20 each side
**Forward Bend & Stretch** - 5

Walk up and down for approximately 30 seconds as your pulse rate reduces.

**Daily Steps:** 10,000 minimum (approximately 3 miles)

**DAY THREE**

### *Limbering Up*

**Toe Touches** - 25
**Arm Rotations** - 20 forwards, 20 backwards
**Lateral Body Bends** - 20 to each side
**Alternate Toe Touches** - 10 to each side
**Running On The Spot** - 105 seconds

### *Core Training*

**Laid Back Kicks** - 19 with each leg
**Roll Backs** - 6
**Arm Lifts** - 19 (6 Left, 6 Right, 7 together)
**Full Sit Ups** - 6

### *Cool Down*

**Lateral Leans** - 20 each side

**Forward Bend & Stretch - 5**

Walk up and down for approximately 30 seconds as your pulse rate reduces.

**Daily Steps:** 10,000 minimum (approximately 3 miles)

**DAY FOUR**

*Limbering Up Only*

**Toe Touches - 25**
**Arm Rotations - 20 forwards, 20 backwards**
**Lateral Body Bends - 20 to each side**
**Alternate Toe Touches - 10 to each side**
**Running On The Spot - 105 seconds**

**Daily Steps:** 10,000 minimum (approximately 3 miles)

**DAY FIVE**

*Limbering Up*

**Toe Touches - 26**
**Arm Rotations - 20 forwards, 20 backwards**
**Lateral Body Bends - 20 to each side**
**Alternate Toe Touches - 10 to each side**
**Running On The Spot - 110 seconds**

*Core Training*

**Laid Back Kicks - 20 with each leg**
**Roll Backs - 7**
**Arm Lifts - 20 (6 Left, 6 Right, 8 together)**
**Full Sit Ups - 7**

*Cool Down*

**Lateral Leans - 20 each side**
**Forward Bend & Stretch - 5**

Walk up and down for approximately 30 seconds as your pulse rate reduces.

**Daily Steps:** 10,000 minimum (approximately 3 miles)


**DAY SIX**

### *Limbering Up*

**Toe Touches** - 26
**Arm Rotations** - 20 forwards, 20 backwards
**Lateral Body Bends** - 20 to each side
**Alternate Toe Touches** - 10 to each side
**Running On The Spot** - 110 seconds

### *Core Training*

**Leg-Passing Knee Pulls** - 9
**Ab Lifts** - 8
**Stepped Push Ups (male)** - 7
**Diamond Push Ups (female)** - 7
**Thigh Squeezes** - 10 sets

### *Cool Down*

**Lateral Leans** - 20 each side
**Forward Bend & Stretch** - 5

Walk up and down for approximately 30 seconds as your pulse rate reduces.

**Daily Steps:** 10,000 minimum (approximately 3 miles)


**DAY SEVEN**

### *Limbering Up*

**Toe Touches** - 27
**Arm Rotations** - 20 forwards, 20 backwards
**Lateral Body Bends** - 20 to each side
**Alternate Toe Touches** - 10 to each side
**Running On The Spot** - 115 seconds

### *Core Training*

**Laid Back Kicks** - 20 with each leg
**Roll Backs** - 7
**Arm Lifts** - 20 (6 Left, 6 Right, 8 together)
**Full Sit Ups** - 7

### *Cool Down*

**Lateral Leans** - 20 each side
**Forward Bend & Stretch** - 5

Walk up and down for approximately 30 seconds as your pulse rate reduces.

**Daily Steps:** 10,000 minimum (approximately 3 miles)

# WEEK SIX

**DAY ONE**

### *Limbering Up*

**Toe Touches** - 27
**Arm Rotations** - 20 forwards, 20 backwards
**Lateral Body Bends** - 20 to each side
**Alternate Toe Touches** - 10 to each side
**Running On The Spot** - 115 seconds

### *Core Training*

**Reverse Curl Ups** - 8
**Hand and Foot** - 11
**Head & Shoulder Lifts** - 13
**Ab Lifts** - 8

### *Cool Down*

**Lateral Leans** - 20 each side
**Forward Bend & Stretch** - 5

Walk up and down for approximately 30 seconds as your pulse rate reduces.

**Daily Steps:** 10,000 minimum (approximately 3 miles)

**DAY TWO**

*Limbering Up*

**Toe Touches** - 28
**Arm Rotations** - 20 forwards, 20 backwards
**Lateral Body Bends** - 20 to each side
**Alternate Toe Touches** - 10 to each side
**Running On The Spot** - 120 seconds

*Core Training*

**Reverse Curl Ups** - 8
**Hand and Foot** - 12
**Head & Shoulder Lifts** - 13
**Ab Lifts** - 8

*Cool Down*

**Lateral Leans** - 20 each side
**Forward Bend & Stretch** - 5

Walk up and down for approximately 30 seconds as your pulse rate reduces.

**Daily Steps:** 10,000 minimum (approximately 3 miles)

**DAY THREE**

*Limbering Up*

**Toe Touches** - 28
**Arm Rotations** - 20 forwards, 20 backwards

**Lateral Body Bends** - 20 to each side
**Alternate Toe Touches** - 10 to each side
**Running On The Spot** - 120 seconds

### *Core Training*

**Stepped Push Ups (male)** - 8
**Diamond Push Ups (female)** - 8
**Lateral Leg Raises** - 19 on each side
**Calf Stretches** - 11
**Leg Hugs**

i)    From an upright standing position step forward approximately 3 feet (nearly one metre) with your right leg

ii)   Lean forward and clasp both hands around your bent knee, holding for 3 seconds, then straighten up and return to an upright position with both legs together.

iii)  Repeat this four more times with your left leg

iv)   Now step forward 3 feet with your right leg, and repeat (ii).

v)    Repeat (iv) twice more, for a total of three for each leg

*Strengthens your thighs, toning your legs and your bottom*

### *Cool Down*

**Lateral Leans** - 20 each side
**Forward Bend & Stretch** - 5

Walk up and down for approximately 30 seconds as your pulse rate reduces.

**Daily Steps:** 10,000 minimum (approximately 3 miles)

**DAY FOUR**

### *Limbering Up Only*

**Toe Touches** - 29
**Arm Rotations** - 20 forwards, 20 backwards
**Lateral Body Bends** - 20 to each side
**Alternate Toe Touches** - 10 to each side
**Running On The Spot** - 120 seconds

**Daily Steps:** 10,000 minimum (approximately 3 miles)

**DAY FIVE**

### *Limbering Up*

**Toe Touches** - 29
**Arm Rotations** - 20 forwards, 20 backwards
**Lateral Body Bends** - 20 to each side
**Alternate Toe Touches** - 10 to each side
**Running On The Spot** - 120 seconds

### *Core Training*

**Stepped Push Ups (male)** - 8
**Diamond Push Ups (female)** - 8
**Lateral Leg Raises** - 20 on each side
**Calf Stretches** - 12
**Leg Hugs** - 5

### *Cool Down*

**Lateral Leans** - 20 each side
**Forward Bend & Stretch** - 5

Walk up and down for approximately 30 seconds as your pulse rate reduces.

**Daily Steps:** 10,000 minimum (approximately 3 miles)

**DAY SIX**

### *Limbering Up*

**Toe Touches** - 30
**Arm Rotations** - 20 forwards, 20 backwards
**Lateral Body Bends** - 20 to each side

**Alternate Toe Touches** – 10 to each side
**Running On The Spot** – 120 seconds

*Core Training*

**Reverse Curl Ups** – 9
**Hand and Foot** – 12
**Head & Shoulder Lifts** – 14
**Ab Lifts** – 8

*Cool Down*

**Lateral Leans** – 20 each side
**Forward Bend & Stretch** – 5

Walk up and down for approximately 30 seconds as your pulse rate reduces.

**Daily Steps:** 10,000 minimum (approximately 3 miles)

**DAY SEVEN**

*Limbering Up*

**Toe Touches** – 30
**Arm Rotations** – 20 forwards, 20 backwards
**Lateral Body Bends** – 20 to each side
**Alternate Toe Touches** – 10 to each side
**Running On The Spot** – 120 seconds

*Core Training*

**Stepped Push Ups (male)** – 9
**Diamond Push Ups (female)** – 9
**Lateral Leg Raises**– 20 on each side
**Calf Stretches** – 12
**Leg Hugs** – 6

*Cool Down*

**Lateral Leans** – 20 each side

**Forward Bend & Stretch** - 5

Walk up and down for approximately 30 seconds as your pulse rate reduces.

**Daily Steps:** 10,000 minimum (approximately 3 miles)


# *WEEK SEVEN*

**DAY ONE**

### *Limbering Up*

**Toe Touches** - 30
**Arm Rotations** - 20 forwards, 20 backwards
**Lateral Body Bends** - 20 to each side
**Alternate Toe Touches** - 10 to each side
**Running On The Spot** - 120 seconds

### *Core Training*

**Hand and Foot** - 13
**Abdominal Strength Training** - 11
**Leg-Passing Knee Pulls** - 9
**Pendulum Leg Swings** - 6

### *Cool Down*

**Lateral Leans** - 20 each side
**Forward Bend & Stretch** - 5

Walk up and down for approximately 30 seconds as your pulse rate reduces.

**Daily Steps:** 10,000 minimum (approximately 3 miles)


**DAY TWO**

### *Limbering Up*

**Toe Touches** - 30
**Arm Rotations** - 20 forwards, 20 backwards
**Lateral Body Bends** - 20 to each side
**Alternate Toe Touches** - 10 to each side
**Running On The Spot** - 120 seconds

### *Core Training*

**Hand and Foot** - 13
**Abdominal Strength Training** - 11
**Leg-Passing Knee Pulls** - 10
**Pendulum Leg Swings** - 7

### *Cool Down*

**Lateral Leans** - 20 each side
**Forward Bend & Stretch** - 5

Walk up and down for approximately 30 seconds as your pulse rate reduces.

**Daily Steps:** 10,000 minimum (approximately 3 miles)

**DAY THREE**

### *Limbering Up*

**Toe Touches** - 30
**Arm Rotations** - 20 forwards, 20 backwards
**Lateral Body Bends** - 20 to each side
**Alternate Toe Touches** - 10 to each side
**Running On The Spot** - 120 seconds

### *Core Training*

**Roll Backs** - 8
**Calf Stretches** - 13
**Thigh Squeezes** - 10 sets
**Full Sit Ups** - 8

### *Cool Down*

**Lateral Leans** - 20 each side
**Forward Bend & Stretch** - 5

Walk up and down for approximately 30 seconds as your pulse rate reduces.

**Daily Steps:** 10,000 minimum (approximately 3 miles)


**DAY FOUR**

### *Limbering Up Only*

**Toe Touches** - 30
**Arm Rotations** - 20 forwards, 20 backwards
**Lateral Body Bends** - 20 to each side
**Alternate Toe Touches** - 10 to each side
**Running On The Spot** - 120 seconds

**Daily Steps:** 10,000 minimum (approximately 3 miles)


**DAY FIVE**

### *Limbering Up*

**Toe Touches** - 30
**Arm Rotations** - 20 forwards, 20 backwards
**Lateral Body Bends** - 20 to each side
**Alternate Toe Touches** - 10 to each side
**Running On The Spot** - 120 seconds

### *Core Training*

**Roll Backs** - 8
**Calf Stretches** - 13
**Thigh Squeezes** - 10 sets
**Full Sit Ups** - 8

### *Cool Down*

**Lateral Leans** - 20 each side

**Forward Bend & Stretch** – 5

Walk up and down for approximately 30 seconds as your pulse rate reduces.

**Daily Steps:** 10,000 minimum (approximately 3 miles)


**DAY SIX**

### *Limbering Up*

**Toe Touches** – 30
**Arm Rotations** – 20 forwards, 20 backwards
**Lateral Body Bends** – 20 to each side
**Alternate Toe Touches** – 10 to each side
**Running On The Spot** – 120 seconds

### *Core Training*

**Hand and Foot** – 14
**Abdominal Strength Training** – 12
**Leg-Passing Knee Pulls** – 10
**Pendulum Leg Swings** – 7

### *Cool Down*

**Lateral Leans** – 20 each side
**Forward Bend & Stretch** – 5

Walk up and down for approximately 30 seconds as your pulse rate reduces.

**Daily Steps:** 10,000 minimum (approximately 3 miles)


**DAY SEVEN**

### *Limbering Up*

**Toe Touches** – 30
**Arm Rotations** – 20 forwards, 20 backwards
**Lateral Body Bends** – 20 to each side

**Alternate Toe Touches** - 10 to each side
**Running On The Spot** - 120 seconds

### *Core Training*

**Roll Backs** - 9
**Calf Stretches** - 14
**Thigh Squeezes** - 10 sets
**Full Sit Ups** - 9

### *Cool Down*

**Lateral Leans** - 20 each side
**Forward Bend & Stretch** - 5

Walk up and down for approximately 30 seconds as your pulse rate reduces.

**Daily Steps:** 10,000 minimum (approximately 3 miles)

# WEEK EIGHT

**DAY ONE**

### *Limbering Up*

**Toe Touches** - 30
**Arm Rotations** - 20 forwards, 20 backwards
**Lateral Body Bends** - 20 to each side
**Alternate Toe Touches** - 10 to each side
**Running On The Spot** - 120 seconds

### *Core Training*

**Laid Back Kicks** - 21 with each leg
**Lateral Leg Raises** - 21 on each side
**Leg Hugs** - 6
**Pendulum Leg Swings** - 8

*Cool Down*

**Lateral Leans** - 20 each side
**Forward Bend & Stretch** - 5

Walk up and down for approximately 30 seconds as your pulse rate reduces.

**Daily Steps:** 10,000 minimum (approximately 3 miles)


**DAY TWO**

*Limbering Up*

**Toe Touches** - 30
**Arm Rotations** - 20 forwards, 20 backwards
**Lateral Body Bends** - 20 to each side
**Alternate Toe Touches** - 10 to each side
**Running On The Spot** - 120 seconds

*Core Training*

**Laid Back Kicks** - 21 with each leg
**Lateral Leg Raises** - 21 on each side
**Leg Hugs** - 7
**Pendulum Leg Swings** - 8

*Cool Down*

**Lateral Leans** - 20 each side
**Forward Bend & Stretch** - 5

Walk up and down for approximately 30 seconds as your pulse rate reduces.

**Daily Steps:** 10,000 minimum (approximately 3 miles)


**DAY THREE**

*Limbering Up*

**Toe Touches** - 30

**Arm Rotations** - 20 forwards, 20 backwards
**Lateral Body Bends** - 20 to each side
**Alternate Toe Touches** - 10 to each side
**Running On The Spot** - 120 seconds

### *Core Training*

**Reverse Curl Ups** - 9
**Head & Shoulder Lifts** - 14
**Ab Lifts** - 8
**Stepped Push Ups (male)** - 9
**Diamond Push Ups (female)** - 9

### *Cool Down*

**Lateral Leans** - 20 each side
**Forward Bend & Stretch** - 5

Walk up and down for approximately 30 seconds as your pulse rate reduces.

**Daily Steps:** 10,000 minimum (approximately 3 miles)

**DAY FOUR**
### *Limbering Up Only*

**Toe Touches** - 30
**Arm Rotations** - 20 forwards, 20 backwards
**Lateral Body Bends** - 20 to each side
**Alternate Toe Touches** - 10 to each side
**Running On The Spot** - 120 seconds

**Daily Steps:** 10,000 minimum (approximately 3 miles)

**DAY FIVE**
### *Limbering Up*

**Toe Touches** - 30
**Arm Rotations** - 20 forwards, 20 backwards

**Lateral Body Bends** - 20 to each side
**Alternate Toe Touches** - 10 to each side
**Running On The Spot** - 120 seconds

### *Core Training*

**Reverse Curl Ups** - 10
**Head & Shoulder Lifts** - 15
**Ab Lifts** - 8
**Stepped Push Ups (male)** - 10
**Diamond Push Ups (female)** - 10

### *Cool Down*

**Lateral Leans** - 20 each side
**Forward Bend & Stretch** - 5

Walk up and down for approximately 30 seconds as your pulse rate reduces.

**Daily Steps:** 10,000 minimum (approximately 3 miles)

**DAY SIX**

### *Limbering Up*

**Toe Touches** - 30
**Arm Rotations** - 20 forwards, 20 backwards
**Lateral Body Bends** - 20 to each side
**Alternate Toe Touches** - 10 to each side
**Running On The Spot** - 120 seconds

### *Core Training*

**Laid Back Kicks** - 22 with each leg
**Lateral Leg Raises** - 22 on each side
**Leg Hugs** - 7
**Pendulum Leg Swings** - 9

### *Cool Down*

**Lateral Leans** - 20 each side
**Forward Bend & Stretch** - 5

Walk up and down for approximately 30 seconds as your pulse rate reduces.

**Daily Steps:** 10,000 minimum (approximately 3 miles)


**DAY SEVEN**

### *Limbering Up*

**Toe Touches** - 30
**Arm Rotations** - 20 forwards, 20 backwards
**Lateral Body Bends** - 20 to each side
**Alternate Toe Touches** - 10 to each side
**Running On The Spot** - 120 seconds

### *Core Training*

**Reverse Curl Ups** - 10
**Head & Shoulder Lifts** - 15
**Ab Lifts** - 8
**Stepped Push Ups (male)** - 10
**Diamond Push Ups (female)** - 10

### *Cool Down*

**Lateral Leans** - 20 each side
**Forward Bend & Stretch** - 5

Walk up and down for approximately 30 seconds as your pulse rate reduces.

**Daily Steps:** 10,000 minimum (approximately 3 miles)


Eight Weeks completed. You should be feeling considerably fitter by now, even though there is plenty of room for improvement. Well done for your persistence. Now it is time to make a final push towards your 12 Week Goal. Review your Weekly

Targets once again. Are you still achieving an 85% strike rate - about 6 days out of 7? Think deeply about your main vision, your long-term goal, and re-set your targets to ensure that it doesn't remain just a pipe dream.

Have you been sticking with the main Exercise Plan? You should have been completing at least an 85% strike rate, and preferably 100% if you are to reap the full rewards. Now there are just 4 weeks left in the initial 12-Week Plan for your greater fitness and over the next 28 days you should be fit enough to exercise every day to take it to the max.

# *WEEK NINE*

**DAY ONE**

### *Limbering Up*

**Toe Touches** - 30
**Arm Rotations** - 20 forwards, 20 backwards
**Lateral Body Bends** - 20 to each side
**Alternate Toe Touches** - 10 to each side
**Running On The Spot** - 120 seconds

### *Core Training*

**Abdominal Strength Training** - 12
**Hand and Foot** - 14
**Arm Lifts** - 21 (7 Left, 7 Right, 7 together)
**Full Sit Ups** - 9

### *Cool Down*

**Lateral Leans** - 20 each side
**Forward Bend & Stretch** - 5

Walk up and down for approximately 30 seconds as your pulse rate reduces.

**Daily Steps:** 10,000 minimum (approximately 3 miles)

**DAY TWO**

*Limbering Up*

**Toe Touches** - 30
**Arm Rotations** - 20 forwards, 20 backwards
**Lateral Body Bends** - 20 to each side
**Alternate Toe Touches** - 10 to each side
**Running On The Spot** - 120 seconds

*Core Training*

**Abdominal Strength Training** - 13
**Hand and Foot** - 15
**Arm Lifts** - 21 (7 Left, 7 Right, 7 together)
**Full Sit Ups** - 10

*Cool Down*

**Lateral Leans** - 20 each side
**Forward Bend & Stretch** - 5

Walk up and down for approximately 30 seconds as your pulse rate reduces.

**Daily Steps:** 10,000 minimum (approximately 3 miles)

**DAY THREE**

*Limbering Up*

**Toe Touches** - 30
**Arm Rotations** - 20 forwards, 20 backwards
**Lateral Body Bends** - 20 to each side
**Alternate Toe Touches** - 10 to each side
**Running On The Spot** - 120 seconds

*Core Training*

**Leg-Passing Knee Pulls** - 11

**Thigh Squeezes** - 10 sets
**Roll Backs** - 9
**Leg Hugs** - 8

*Cool Down*

**Lateral Leans** - 20 each side
**Forward Bend & Stretch** - 5

Walk up and down for approximately 30 seconds as your pulse rate reduces.

**Daily Steps:** 10,000 minimum (approximately 3 miles)

**DAY FOUR**

*Limbering Up*

**Toe Touches** - 30
**Arm Rotations** - 20 forwards, 20 backwards
**Lateral Body Bends** - 20 to each side
**Alternate Toe Touches** - 10 to each side
**Running On The Spot** - 120 seconds

*Core Training*

**Leg-Passing Knee Pulls** - 11
**Thigh Squeezes** - 10 sets
**Roll Backs** - 9
**Leg Hugs** - 8

*Cool Down*

**Lateral Leans** - 20 each side
**Forward Bend & Stretch** - 5

Walk up and down for approximately 30 seconds as your pulse rate reduces.

**Daily Steps:** 10,000 minimum (approximately 3 miles)

**DAY FIVE**

*Limbering Up*

**Toe Touches** - 30
**Arm Rotations** - 20 forwards, 20 backwards
**Lateral Body Bends** - 20 to each side
**Alternate Toe Touches** - 10 to each side
**Running On The Spot** - 120 seconds

*Core Training*

**Abdominal Strength Training** - 13
**Hand and Foot** - 15
**Arm Lifts** - 22 (7 Left, 7 Right, 8 together)
**Full Sit Ups** - 10

*Cool Down*

**Lateral Leans** - 20 each side
**Forward Bend & Stretch** - 5

Walk up and down for approximately 30 seconds as your pulse rate reduces.

**Daily Steps:** 10,000 minimum (approximately 3 miles)

**DAY SIX**

*Limbering Up*

**Toe Touches** - 30
**Arm Rotations** - 20 forwards, 20 backwards
**Lateral Body Bends** - 20 to each side
**Alternate Toe Touches** - 10 to each side
**Running On The Spot** - 120 seconds

*Core Training*

**Leg-Passing Knee Pulls** - 12
**Thigh Squeezes** - 10 sets
**Roll Backs** - 9

**Leg Hugs** - 9

### *Cool Down*

**Lateral Leans** - 20 each side
**Forward Bend & Stretch** - 5

Walk up and down for approximately 30 seconds as your pulse rate reduces.

**Daily Steps:** 10,000 minimum (approximately 3 miles)


**DAY SEVEN**

### *Limbering Up*

**Toe Touches** - 30
**Arm Rotations** - 20 forwards, 20 backwards
**Lateral Body Bends** - 20 to each side
**Alternate Toe Touches** - 10 to each side
**Running On The Spot** - 120 seconds

### *Core Training*

**Abdominal Strength Training** - 14
**Hand and Foot** - 16
**Arm Lifts** - 22 (7 Left, 7 Right, 8 together)
**Full Sit Ups** - 11

### *Cool Down*

**Lateral Leans** - 20 each side
**Forward Bend & Stretch** - 5

Walk up and down for approximately 30 seconds as your pulse rate reduces.

**Daily Steps:** 10,000 minimum (approximately 3 miles)

# *WEEK TEN*

**DAY ONE**

### *Limbering Up*

**Toe Touches** - 30
**Arm Rotations** - 20 forwards, 20 backwards
**Lateral Body Bends** - 20 to each side
**Alternate Toe Touches** - 10 to each side
**Running On The Spot** - 120 seconds

### *Core Training*

**Laid Back Kicks** - 22 with each leg
**Head & Shoulder Lifts** - 16
**Calf Stretches** - 14
**Stepped Push Ups (male)** - 11
**Diamond Push Ups (female)** - 11

### *Cool Down*

**Lateral Leans** - 20 each side
**Forward Bend & Stretch** - 5

Walk up and down for approximately 30 seconds as your pulse rate reduces.

**Daily Steps:** 10,000 minimum (approximately 3 miles)

**DAY TWO**

### *Limbering Up*

**Toe Touches** - 30
**Arm Rotations** - 20 forwards, 20 backwards
**Lateral Body Bends** - 20 to each side
**Alternate Toe Touches** - 10 to each side
**Running On The Spot** - 120 seconds

### *Core Training*

**Laid Back Kicks** - 23 with each leg
**Head & Shoulder Lifts** - 16
**Calf Stretches** - 15
**Stepped Push Ups (male)** - 11
**Diamond Push Ups (female)** - 11

### *Cool Down*

**Lateral Leans** - 20 each side
**Forward Bend & Stretch** - 5

Walk up and down for approximately 30 seconds as your pulse rate reduces.

**Daily Steps:** 10,000 minimum (approximately 3 miles)

**DAY THREE**

### *Limbering Up*

**Toe Touches** - 30
**Arm Rotations** - 20 forwards, 20 backwards
**Lateral Body Bends** - 20 to each side
**Alternate Toe Touches** - 10 to each side
**Running On The Spot** - 120 seconds

### *Core Training*

**Abdominal Strength Training** - 14
**Reverse Curl Ups** - 11
**Lateral Leg Raises** - 22 on each side
**Pendulum Leg Swings** - 9

### *Cool Down*

**Lateral Leans** - 20 each side
**Forward Bend & Stretch** - 5

Walk up and down for approximately 30 seconds as your pulse rate reduces.

**Daily Steps:** 10,000 minimum (approximately 3 miles)


**DAY FOUR**

### *Limbering Up*

**Toe Touches** - 30
**Arm Rotations** - 20 forwards, 20 backwards
**Lateral Body Bends** - 20 to each side
**Alternate Toe Touches** - 10 to each side
**Running On The Spot** - 120 seconds

### *Core Training*

**Abdominal Strength Training** - 15
**Reverse Curl Ups** - 11
**Lateral Leg Raises** - 23 on each side
**Pendulum Leg Swings** - 10

### *Cool Down*

**Lateral Leans** - 20 each side
**Forward Bend & Stretch** - 5

Walk up and down for approximately 30 seconds as your pulse rate reduces.

**Daily Steps:** 10,000 minimum (approximately 3 miles)


**DAY FIVE**

### *Limbering Up*

**Toe Touches** - 30
**Arm Rotations** - 20 forwards, 20 backwards
**Lateral Body Bends** - 20 to each side
**Alternate Toe Touches** - 10 to each side
**Running On The Spot** - 120 seconds

### *Core Training*

**Laid Back Kicks** - 23 with each leg
**Head & Shoulder Lifts** - 17
**Calf Stretches** - 15
**Stepped Push Ups (male)** - 12
**Diamond Push Ups (female)** - 12

### *Cool Down*

**Lateral Leans** - 20 each side
**Forward Bend & Stretch** - 5

Walk up and down for approximately 30 seconds as your pulse rate reduces.

**Daily Steps:** 10,000 minimum (approximately 3 miles)

**DAY SIX**
### *Limbering Up*

**Toe Touches** - 30
**Arm Rotations** - 20 forwards, 20 backwards
**Lateral Body Bends** - 20 to each side
**Alternate Toe Touches** - 10 to each side
**Running On The Spot** - 120 seconds

### *Core Training*

**Abdominal Strength Training** - 15
**Reverse Curl Ups** - 12
**Lateral Leg Raises** - 23 on each side
**Pendulum Leg Swings** - 10

### *Cool Down*

**Lateral Leans** - 20 each side
**Forward Bend & Stretch** - 5

Walk up and down for approximately 30 seconds as your pulse rate reduces.

**Daily Steps:** 10,000 minimum (approximately 3 miles)

**DAY SEVEN**

*Limbering Up*

**Toe Touches** - 30
**Arm Rotations** - 20 forwards, 20 backwards
**Lateral Body Bends** - 20 to each side
**Alternate Toe Touches** - 10 to each side
**Running On The Spot** - 120 seconds

*Core Training*

**Laid Back Kicks** - 24 with each leg
**Head & Shoulder Lifts** - 17
**Calf Stretches** - 15
**Stepped Push Ups (male)** - 12
**Diamond Push Ups (female)** - 12

*Cool Down*

**Lateral Leans** - 20 each side
**Forward Bend & Stretch** - 5

Walk up and down for approximately 30 seconds as your pulse rate reduces.

**Daily Steps:** 10,000 minimum (approximately 3 miles)

# WEEK ELEVEN

**DAY ONE**

*Limbering Up*

**Toe Touches** - 30
**Arm Rotations** - 20 forwards, 20 backwards
**Lateral Body Bends** - 20 to each side
**Alternate Toe Touches** - 10 to each side

**Running On The Spot** - 120 seconds

### *Core Training*

**Roll Backs** - 9
**Leg Hugs** - 9
**Arm Lifts** - 23 (7 Left, 7 Right, 9 together)
**Stepped Push Ups (male)** - 13
**Diamond Push Ups (female)** - 13

### *Cool Down*

**Lateral Leans** - 20 each side
**Forward Bend & Stretch** - 5

Walk up and down for approximately 30 seconds as your pulse rate reduces.

**Daily Steps:** 10,000 minimum (approximately 3 miles)

**DAY TWO**

### *Limbering Up*

**Toe Touches** - 30
**Arm Rotations** - 20 forwards, 20 backwards
**Lateral Body Bends** - 20 to each side
**Alternate Toe Touches** - 10 to each side
**Running On The Spot** - 120 seconds

### *Core Training*

**Roll Backs** - 9
**Leg Hugs** - 10
**Arm Lifts** - 23 (7 Left, 7 Right, 9 together)
**Stepped Push Ups (male)** - 13
**Diamond Push Ups (female)** - 13

### *Cool Down*

**Lateral Leans** - 20 each side

**Forward Bend & Stretch** - 5

Walk up and down for approximately 30 seconds as your pulse rate reduces.

**Daily Steps:** 10,000 minimum (approximately 3 miles)


**DAY THREE**
### *Limbering Up*

**Toe Touches** - 30
**Arm Rotations** - 20 forwards, 20 backwards
**Lateral Body Bends** - 20 to each side
**Alternate Toe Touches** - 10 to each side
**Running On The Spot** - 120 seconds

### *Core Training*

**Laid Back Kicks** - 24 with each leg
**Hand and Foot** - 16
**Ab Lifts** - 8
**Full Sit Ups** - 11

### *Cool Down*

**Lateral Leans** - 20 each side
**Forward Bend & Stretch** - 5

Walk up and down for approximately 30 seconds as your pulse rate reduces.

**Daily Steps:** 10,000 minimum (approximately 3 miles)


**DAY FOUR**
### *Limbering Up*

**Toe Touches** - 30
**Arm Rotations** - 20 forwards, 20 backwards
**Lateral Body Bends** - 20 to each side
**Alternate Toe Touches** - 10 to each side

**Running On The Spot** - 120 seconds

### *Core Training*

**Laid Back Kicks** - 25 with each leg
**Hand and Foot** - 17
**Ab Lifts** - 8
**Full Sit Ups** - 12

### *Cool Down*

**Lateral Leans** - 20 each side
**Forward Bend & Stretch** - 5

Walk up and down for approximately 30 seconds as your pulse rate reduces.

**Daily Steps:** 10,000 minimum (approximately 3 miles)

DAY FIVE

### *Limbering Up*

**Toe Touches** - 30
**Arm Rotations** - 20 forwards, 20 backwards
**Lateral Body Bends** - 20 to each side
**Alternate Toe Touches** - 10 to each side
**Running On The Spot** - 120 seconds

### *Core Training*

**Roll Backs** - 9
**Leg Hugs** - 10
**Arm Lifts** - 24 (8 Left, 8 Right, 8 together)
**Stepped Push Ups (male)** - 14
**Diamond Push Ups (female)** - 14

### *Cool Down*

**Lateral Leans** - 20 each side
**Forward Bend & Stretch** - 5

Walk up and down for approximately 30 seconds as your pulse rate reduces.

**Daily Steps:** 10,000 minimum (approximately 3 miles)


## DAY SIX

### *Limbering Up*

**Toe Touches** - 30
**Arm Rotations** - 20 forwards, 20 backwards
**Lateral Body Bends** - 20 to each side
**Alternate Toe Touches** - 10 to each side
**Running On The Spot** - 120 seconds


### *Core Training*

**Laid Back Kicks** - 25 with each leg
**Hand and Foot** - 17
**Ab Lifts** - 8
**Full Sit Ups** - 12


### *Cool Down*

**Lateral Leans** - 20 each side
**Forward Bend & Stretch** - 5

Walk up and down for approximately 30 seconds as your pulse rate reduces.

**Daily Steps:** 10,000 minimum (approximately 3 miles)


## DAY SEVEN

### *Limbering Up*

**Toe Touches** - 30
**Arm Rotations** - 20 forwards, 20 backwards
**Lateral Body Bends** - 20 to each side
**Alternate Toe Touches** - 10 to each side
**Running On The Spot** - 120 seconds

### *Core Training*

**Roll Backs** – 9
**Leg Hugs** – 11
**Arm Lifts** – 24 (8 Left, 8 Right, 8 together)
**Stepped Push Ups (male)** – 14
**Diamond Push Ups (female)** – 14

### *Cool Down*

**Lateral Leans** – 20 each side
**Forward Bend & Stretch** – 5

Walk up and down for approximately 30 seconds as your pulse rate reduces.

**Daily Steps:** 10,000 minimum (approximately 3 miles)

# WEEK TWELVE

**DAY ONE**

### *Limbering Up*

**Toe Touches** – 30
**Arm Rotations** – 20 forwards, 20 backwards
**Lateral Body Bends** – 20 to each side
**Alternate Toe Touches** – 10 to each side
**Running On The Spot** – 120 seconds

### *Core Training*

**Leg-Passing Knee Pulls** – 12
**Pendulum Leg Swings** – 11
**Head & Shoulder Lifts** – 18
**Thigh Squeezes** – 10 sets

### *Cool Down*

**Lateral Leans** - 20 each side
**Forward Bend & Stretch** - 5

Walk up and down for approximately 30 seconds as your pulse rate reduces.

**Daily Steps:** 10,000 minimum (approximately 3 miles)


**DAY TWO**

*Limbering Up*

**Toe Touches** - 30
**Arm Rotations** - 20 forwards, 20 backwards
**Lateral Body Bends** - 20 to each side
**Alternate Toe Touches** - 10 to each side
**Running On The Spot** - 120 seconds

*Core Training*

**Leg-Passing Knee Pulls** - 13
**Pendulum Leg Swings** - 11
**Head & Shoulder Lifts** - 18
**Thigh Squeezes** - 10 sets

*Cool Down*

**Lateral Leans** - 20 each side
**Forward Bend & Stretch** - 5

Walk up and down for approximately 30 seconds as your pulse rate reduces.

**Daily Steps:** 10,000 minimum (approximately 3 miles)


**DAY THREE**

*Limbering Up*

**Toe Touches** - 30
**Arm Rotations** - 20 forwards, 20 backwards

**Lateral Body Bends** - 20 to each side
**Alternate Toe Touches** - 10 to each side
**Running On The Spot** - 120 seconds

### *Core Training*

**Abdominal Strength Training** - 16
**Roll Backs** - 9
**Arm Lifts** - 25 (8 Left, 8 Right, 9 together)
**Leg Hugs** - 11

### *Cool Down*

**Lateral Leans** - 20 each side
**Forward Bend & Stretch** - 5

Walk up and down for approximately 30 seconds as your pulse rate reduces.

**Daily Steps:** 10,000 minimum (approximately 3 miles)

**DAY FOUR**

### *Limbering Up*

**Toe Touches** - 30
**Arm Rotations** - 20 forwards, 20 backwards
**Lateral Body Bends** - 20 to each side
**Alternate Toe Touches** - 10 to each side
**Running On The Spot** - 120 seconds

### *Core Training*

**Abdominal Strength Training**- 16
**Roll Backs** - 9
**Arm Lifts** - 25 (8 Left, 8 Right, 9 together)
**Leg Hugs** - 12

### *Cool Down*

**Lateral Leans** - 20 each side

**Forward Bend & Stretch** - 5

Walk up and down for approximately 30 seconds as your pulse rate reduces.

**Daily Steps:** 10,000 minimum (approximately 3 miles)


**DAY FIVE**

### *Limbering Up*

**Toe Touches** - 30
**Arm Rotations** - 20 forwards, 20 backwards
**Lateral Body Bends** - 20 to each side
**Alternate Toe Touches** - 10 to each side
**Running On The Spot** - 120 seconds

### *Core Training*

**Leg-Passing Knee Pulls** - 13
**Pendulum Leg Swings** - 12
**Head & Shoulder Lifts** - 19
**Thigh Squeezes** - 10 sets

### *Cool Down*

**Lateral Leans** - 20 each side
**Forward Bend & Stretch** - 5

Walk up and down for approximately 30 seconds as your pulse rate reduces.

**Daily Steps:** 10,000 minimum (approximately 3 miles)


**DAY SIX**

### *Limbering Up*

**Toe Touches** - 30
**Arm Rotations** - 20 forwards, 20 backwards
**Lateral Body Bends** - 20 to each side
**Alternate Toe Touches** - 10 to each side

**Running On The Spot** - 120 seconds

### *Core Training*

**Abdominal Strength Training** - 16
**Roll Backs** - 9
**Arm Lifts** - 26 (8 Left, 8 Right, 10 together)
**Leg Hugs** - 12

### *Cool Down*

**Lateral Leans** - 20 each side
**Forward Bend & Stretch** - 5

Walk up and down for approximately 30 seconds as your pulse rate reduces.

**Daily Steps:** 10,000 minimum (approximately 3 miles)

**DAY SEVEN**

### *Limbering Up*

**Toe Touches** - 30
**Arm Rotations** - 20 forwards, 20 backwards
**Lateral Body Bends** - 20 to each side
**Alternate Toe Touches** - 10 to each side
**Running On The Spot** - 120 seconds

### *Core Training*

**Leg-Passing Knee Pulls** - 14
**Pendulum Leg Swings** - 12
**Head & Shoulder Lifts** - 19
**Thigh Squeezes** - 10 sets

### *Cool Down*

**Lateral Leans** - 20 each side
**Forward Bend & Stretch** - 5

Walk up and down for approximately 30 seconds as your pulse rate reduces.

**Daily Steps:** 10,000 minimum (approximately 3 miles)

# *IS THIS THE END?*

Twelve Weeks completed! Have you met your targets? What types of improvement have you experienced? Whether it is a trimmer waistline, a buoyant spring in your step or perhaps a far easier climb up nearby hills, I would love to know what has improved for you so far. If you have reached your target, or moved significantly in that direction then please let me know.  If the opposite is true then also let me know. Your feedback is important.

I hope that the amazing progress you have made over the last 12 weeks will have inspired you to continue. You have now mastered all the exercises in this 12 Week Exercise Plan, but there is no reason to stop right here. You now have the keys to a fitter future. You have taken it for a test drive and now you own your future.

So where do you go from here?

Remember your Vision, your grand design for where you want to be in the coming months or years? You have now progressed 12 weeks closer to it, positively and in control of your future.

So take time out to step back and review your main target for the coming 12 weeks. Make this day a Rest Day after your exertions over the last four weeks, and think about setting a challenging target to reach 12 weeks from now. Then set some new weekly targets which you estimate will help you to get there.

Continue the same sequence of exercises, taking a rest day once a week except for occasions when you need extra momentum. Here is a guide to the maximum recommended level for each exercise – which I term The Maintenance Level - to maintain your fitness now and far into the future. I continue to commit myself to these daily, almost without fail, and quite often to a greater level when the mood takes me. Bearing in mind that I am reaching my mid-sixties as I write this, I would expect that the level of exercise set out here should be pretty easy for someone as healthy as you are now becoming in your fit forties.

## The Maintenance Level

**Alternate Toe Touches** - 20 to each side
**Arm Rotations** - 20 forwards, 20 backwards

**Lateral Body Bends** - 20 to each side
**Running On The Spot** - 120 seconds
**Toe Touches** - 30

**Ab Lifts** – 8
**Abdominal Strength Training** – 16
**Arm Lifts** – 36 with each arm
**Calf Stretches** - 15
**Full Sit Ups** – 25
**Hand and Foot** - 20
**Head & Shoulder Lifts** - 25
**Laid Back Kicks** - 35 with each leg
**Lateral Leg Raises** - 30 with each leg
**Leg Hugs** - 15 with each leg
**Leg-Passing Knee Pulls** – 15
**Pendulum Leg Swings** - 20
**Stepped Push Ups (male)** - 20
**Diamond Push Ups (female)** - 15
**Reverse Curl Ups** - 15
**Roll Backs** – 9
**Thigh Squeezes** - 10 sets

**Forward Bend & Stretch** - 5
**Lateral Leans** - 20 each side

When you have reached the Maintenance Level then your fitness should be assured. Even if you miss a day or two of these routine exercises every now and then. Even if you succumb to a period of excessive over-indulgence at certain times of the year. That shouldn't be a problem.

However, although your fitness won't desert you without some serious neglect on your part, it will certainly be more difficult to regain it after a few weeks without proper exercise. On other occasions you may put on a few pounds if you have over-indulged just that bit too much. It will be quite easy to shed with a few days of a lower calorie intake, in proportion to whatever has led to the excess, coupled with a little extra exercise over and above the maintenance level.

Beware though. Neglecting your fitness for too long will make it easier to put off the day when you pick it up again, and make it more difficult when you begin. Please don't let it happen to you now that you have come so far. If you feel that you may need support to keep up the momentum then I recommend joining the Easy Fitness Group, which is discussed a little further on.

Easy Fitness is easy. It only becomes more difficult when you allow your fitness level to drop. You don't want to start at Week One again. Trust me, I know!

Now that your first 12 weeks are complete, you are well set for a better, fitter, future. However, you don't need to go there alone. Let me help you maintain that fitness level, encourage you to continue when your resolve may be weakening, and even show you how to progress to the next level. You are on the right path to a much healthier lifestyle, and I hope you will agree with me that setting out on this journey and arriving at this staging post has been much easier than you imagined.

You should be able to continue along this path on your own, keeping up the same sequence of exercises to the maximum recommended level. From this point you can reach 50 years old and still have the body of a 40 year old. It would certainly be a shame to go backwards from here, as I myself did when I reached the latter half of my forties. If you would like to join me in the Easy Fitness group then we can continue on this journey together. This is the end of the book, but it need not stop right here.

Remember, when you turn 50 your muscles start wasting away – if you don't use them. So keep it up, and if you need support in continuing your progress then I am here for you.

If you have any questions about *Easy Fitness for Over 40s*, here's my personal email address, and feel free to use it: ChrisMorris6217@gmail.com

For more fitness tips and advice, and extensions to this course, please pay a regular visit to https://easyfitnessfor life.net